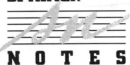

SPRINGHOUSE

NOTES

HEALTH ASSESSMENT

Elizabeth D. Metzgar, RNC, MPH, FNP

Ms. Metzgar, a coauthor of this book, is an Assistant Professor at Montana State University, Missoula, and Co-Project Director of the university's Family Nursing Clinic. She earned her BSN from Ohio State University, Columbus, and received her MPH from the University of Michigan, Ann Arbor. She is also a certified family nurse practitioner. Ms. Metzgar is a member of the American Nurses' Association, the National League for Nursing, the American Public Health Association, and Sigma Theta Tau.

Karen A. Stinger, RNC, MS, PNP

Ms. Stinger, a coauthor of this book, is an Assistant Professor at Montana State University, Missoula, and Co-Project Director of the university's Family Nursing Clinic. She received her BSN from Eastern Washington University, Cheney, and earned her MS from Arizona State University, Tempe. She is also a certified pediatric nurse practitioner. Ms. Stinger is a member of the International Association for Care of Children's Health and Sigma Theta Tau.

Linda L. Grabbe, RN, MN, CCRN

Ms. Grabbe, the reviewer of this book, is a Clinical Instructor at the University of North Carolina at Chapel Hill. She earned her BSN from the University of Hawaii at Manoa, and received her MN from Emory University, Atlanta. She is also a critical-care registered nurse. Ms. Grabbe is a member of the American Nurses' Association, the American Association of Critical-Care Nurses, the American Association of Neuroscience Nurses, and Sigma Theta Tau.

Springhouse Publishing Company
Springhouse, Pennsylvania

STAFF FOR THIS VOLUME

CLINICAL STAFF

Clinical Director
Barbara McVan, RN

Clinical Editors
Lynne Atkinson, RN, BSN, CEN
Joan E. Mason, RN, EdM
Diane Schweisguth, RN, BSN, CCRN, CEN

ADVISORY BOARD

Mildred Wernet Boyd, RN, BSN, MSN
Assistant Professor, Essex Community College,
Baltimore

Dorothy Brooten, PhD, FAAN
Chairperson, Health Care of Women and
Childbearing Section, Director of Graduate Perinatal
Nursing, University of Pennsylvania School of
Nursing, Philadelphia

Lillian S. Brunner, MSN, ScD, LittD, FAAN
Nurse/Author, Brunner Associates, Inc., Berwyn, Pa.

Irma J. D'Antonio, RN, PhD
Professor and Chairperson, Department of Nursing,
Mount St. Mary's College, Los Angeles

Kathleen Dracup, RN, DNSc, FAAN
Associate Professor, School of Nursing, University of
California, Los Angeles, Los Angeles

Cecile A. Lengacher, RN, PhD
Director of the Division of Nursing and Health
Sciences, Manatee Junior College, Bradenton, Fla.

Barbara Tower, RN, MSN, CCRN
Assistant Professor, Essex Community College,
Baltimore

PUBLICATION STAFF

Executive Director, Editorial
Stanley Loeb

Executive Director, Creative Services
Jean Robinson

Design
John Hubbard (art director), Stephanie Peters
(associate art director), Jacalyn Bove Facciolo,
Julie Carleton Barlow

Editing
Donna L. Hilton (acquisitions), Kathy E. Goldberg,
Patricia McKeown, David Prout

Copy Editing
David Moreau (manager), Edith McMahon
(supervisor), Nick Anastasio, Keith de Pinho, Diane
Labus, Doris Weinstock, Debra Young

Art Production
Robert Perry (manager), Anna Brindisi, Christopher
Buckley, Loretta Caruso, Donald Knauss, Christina
McKinley, Mark Marcin, Robert Wieder

Typography
David Kosten (manager), Diane Paluba (assistant
manager), Joyce Rossi Biletz, Alicia Dempsey,
Brenda Mayer, Nancy Wirs

Manufacturing
Deborah Meiris (manager)

Project Coordination
Aline S. Miller (supervisor), Maureen Carmichael

Library of Congress Cataloging-in-Publication Data

Metzgar, Elizabeth D.
  Health assessment.

  (Springhouse notes)
  Includes bibliographies and index.
  1. Physical diagnosis—Outlines, syllabi, etc.
2. Nursing—Outlines, syllabi, etc. I. Stinger,
Karen A. II. Grabbe, Linda L. III. Title.
  IV. Series. [DNLM: Health.   WB 141.4 M596h]
RT48.5.M48   1988   616.07'54   87-18081
ISBN 0-87434-115-9

Contents

How to Use Springhouse Notes

Today, more than ever, nursing students face enormous time pressures. Nursing education has become more sophisticated, increasing the difficulties students have with studying efficiently and keeping pace.

The need for a comprehensive, well-designed series of study aids is great, which is why we've produced Springhouse Notes...to meet that need. Springhouse Notes provide essential course material in outline form, enabling the nursing student to study more effectively, improve understanding, achieve higher test scores, and get better grades.

Key features appear throughout each book, making the information more accessible and easier to remember.
- **Learning Objectives.** These objectives precede each section in the book to help the student evaluate knowledge before and after study.
- **Key Points.** Highlighted in color throughout the book, these points provide a way to quickly review critical information. Key points may include:
—a cardinal sign or symptom of a disorder
—the most current or popular theory about a topic
—a distinguishing characteristic of a disorder
—the most important step of a process
—a critical assessment component
—a crucial nursing intervention
—the most widely used or successful therapy or treatment.
- **Points to Remember.** This information, found at the end of each section, summarizes the section in capsule form.
- **Glossary.** Difficult, frequently used, or sometimes misunderstood terms are defined for the student at the end of each section.

Remember: Springhouse Notes are learning tools designed to *help* you. They are not intended for use as a primary information source. They should never substitute for class attendance, text reading, or classroom note taking.

This book, Health Assessment, begins with a general overview of the subject, then continues with physical, family, and social history taking; review of systems; and assessment of current health status. After that, each body system or body area assessment covers anatomy and physiology, and procedures and normal findings for each assessment technique (as appropriate)—inspection, auscultation, palpation, and percussion.

Overview of Health Assessment

Learning Objectives

After studying this section, the reader should be able to:

• Identify major components of health assessment from a theoretical perspective.

• Describe the relationship between nursing process and health assessment.

• Identify the major components of a subjective data base.

• Identify the major components of an objective data base.

• Identify principles for collecting and recording health assessment data.

I. Overview of Health Assessment

A. Major theoretical perspectives underlying health assessment
1. Considers the relationship between individual clients and their social environment
2. Considers client as someone affected by many subsystems: physiological, psychological, social, economic, cultural, and environmental
3. Demonstrates how each subsystem affects client
4. Encourages the health care provider to approach client as a whole person

B. Major theoretical perspectives used in this text
1. Systems theory
   a. A system is a set of interrelated, interdependent parts
   b. All living systems are open systems, affected by external as well as internal forces
   c. A system tries to reduce tension and achieve homeostasis between external and internal forces
   d. The whole system is greater than the sum of its parts
2. Holism
   a. An individual differs from and exceeds the sum of his/her parts
   b. Body, mind, and spirit are interdependent and interact dynamically with the environmment
   c. Responses to life processes are complex, integrated, and individualized. Growth and development, along with personal history, socio-cultural background, and economic factors, all affect data collection and data analysis
3. Developmental theory
   a. Growth, maturation, and change are inherent to life
   b. Development is a lifelong, evolutionary process of change in structure, thought, and behavior that results from physical and mental maturation, learning, and experience and leads to a more advanced level of maturity and integration

C. Psychosocial considerations in health assessment
1. General
   a. A person is unique, but functions within the broader contexts of his/her sex, genetic potential, developmental stage, family system, cultural/ethnic background, and socio-economic status
   b. A physical symptom or finding doesn't exist in a vacuum; it is mediated by age, race, culture, environment, family, mood, and availability of health care
   c. Even initial impressions, such as dress, mannerisms, behavior, and physical appearance, are mediated by psychosocial factors. Observation and communication are required to locate a datum within its larger frame of reference

2. Developmental
   a. Development occurs in orderly, predictable stages from birth to death, but procession from one stage to the next depends on the interaction of maturational potential with the social and physical environment
   b. Growth and development affect but do not change behavior
   c. During critical growth periods, a system's disorganization makes it particularly susceptible to environmental effects
   d. Development of physical, cognitive, emotional, and social competencies occur simultaneously and interdependently
3. Racial/Cultural/Religious
   a. Culture determines a person's definition of health and illness and response to the health/illness continuum
   b. Many diseases or risks for acquiring disease are racially determined
   c. Knowledge of cultural factors aids in interpreting an individual's development and behavior
   d. Decisions about seeking health care are culturally mediated
   e. Nutritional patterns may be set by cultural/religious beliefs
4. Environmental
   a. Environments include factors that affect physical health: air pollutants, water pollutants, noise hazards, safety hazards
   b. Environments affect psychological well-being by providing or lacking adequate space or a relaxing atmosphere
5. Family/Social
   a. The family is the primary unit for organizing, performing, and securing health behavior and care
   b. Health promoting/protecting beliefs and behaviors are learned from the family or significant social system: for example, beliefs about hygiene, rest pattern, diet, exercise, and self-care
   c. Genetic factors are inherited
   d. Behavior is defined and interpreted within the context of social norms
6. Economic/Occupational
   a. Economic level affects self-concept and self-confidence in interactions with society
   b. Access to health care, availability of insurance, and decisions about when to seek care depend on economic level
   c. Occupations may involve safety hazards, sensory strains, psychological stress
7. Psychological
   a. The relationship of stress to a variety of physical illnesses is increasingly well documented
   b. Stress is also necessary for growth and development and can positively affect adaptation
   c. Emotional states affect a person's ability to cope, to participate in care, to change behaviors, and to utilize supportive resources
   d. The client's ability to interact positively with caregivers depends in part on his or her mental/temperamental/personality makeup

8. Psychosocial considerations for the caregiver
   a. Caregivers must know how their own pyschosocial history affects their ability to assist clients
   b. Caregivers must understand the effect that their knowledge, experience, and comfort level have on interactions with clients and on the sense of self-confidence that they must communicate

D. Major components of health assessment
1. Nursing history: specific data about self related to nurse by client or significant other; major subjective data source
2. Physical assessment: inspection, palpation, auscultation, and percussion to examine body for normal anatomic and physiologic findings; major objective data source
3. Screening: procedure used by the nurse to assess the condition of a system, such as developmental or vision screening
4. Summary of health assessment results: narrative that describes subjective and objective findings and lists nursing diagnoses

E. Overview of subjective data base
1. Purposes of health history
   a. Provides ongoing record of client's well-being
   b. Provides baseline data for focusing physical assessment
   c. Enables nurse to assess client's total state of health and formulate nursing diagnoses
   d. Provides mechanism to evaluate the effectiveness of nursing care
2. Factors critical to data collection process
   a. Appraising reliability of the informant
   b. Establishing rapport and trust
   c. Discussing confidentiality
   d. Providing private, comfortable surroundings
   e. Establishing realistic time frame
   f. Keeping interactions free from judgments, bias, and imposition of values on the client
   g. Establishing the client's goals for the interview
   h. Assessing verbal and nonverbal behaviors of client
3. Major components of health history
   a. Biographic/demographic information
   b. Current health status
   c. Health history
   d. Family history
   e. Personal social history
   f. Health promotion and protection behaviors
   g. Review of systems

F. Effective communication techniques for nurse obtaining a health history
 1. Factors affecting communication process
    a. Culture of client
    b. Language; primary spoken language of client
    c. Education level of client
    d. Sensory impairments
 2. Nonverbal techniques
    a. Appropriate eye contact
    b. Open body posture; e.g., limbs extended, arms relaxed rather than tense against body
    c. Neutral facial expression
    d. Appropriate use of touch to convey empathy
    e. Dress and appearance appropriate to the socio-cultural milieu of the client
    f. Awareness of congruence between client's verbal and nonverbal behavior
    g. Awareness of client's body language when it contradicts what client says
 3. Effective verbal techniques
    a. Being aware of how nurse's personality and method of sequencing questions influences client response
    b. Using common language and avoiding medical jargon
    c. Encouraging clients to verbalize by using periods of silence
    d. Beginning interview with least personal questions first
    e. Using effective interviewing techniques and not blocking verbal communication

G. Effective interviewing techniques for collecting subjective data
 1. Using open-ended questions for majority of history
    a. Avoids yes and no responses
    b. Elicits comparative and descriptive responses
    c. Provides data about alertness, cognitive processing, and attitude
    d. May result in rambling or withholding specific information about a vital point
    e. Includes such statements as "Tell me the purpose of your visit today."
 2. Using closed-ended questions
    a. Yields one or two word responses
    b. Provides specific information
    c. Is appropriate for educationally disadvantaged client or those who speak little English
    d. Is occasionally useful for focusing a rambling client
 3. Using examples
    a. Clarifies meaning to create mutual understanding
    b. Provides the opportunity to raise such questions as "Was the mole as big as a dime?"
 4. Providing general leads
    a. Permits client to direct discussion
    b. Covers areas of personal importance to client

5. Repeating or restating
   a. Ensures accuracy
   b. Lets client know that he has effectively communicated
   c. Includes such questions as "Do you mean you take your heart medication every 8 hours?"
6. Clarifying
   a. Assures mutual understanding of health behavior or symptom
   b. If repeated attempts at clarification are unsuccessful, nurse should use secondary data source such as friends or relatives
   c. Use such statements as "I'm not certain I understand what you mean."
7. Offering reality
   a. Useful for dealing with misperceptions about health status or health care
   b. Uses such statements as "I'm not sure I can agree with that."
8. Putting the implied into words
   a. Helps nurse avoid inferences
   b. Ensures accurate interpretation of client's meaning
   c. Involves such scenarios as: Client, "My student role makes family life difficult sometimes." Nurse, "Do you get to spend enough time with your children?"
9. Seeking evaluation
   a. Allows client to take part in decisions about health care
   b. May help client comply with therapeutic regimen
   c. Includes such questions as "How will this plan affect your routine?"
10. Providing information
    a. Offers teaching opportunities
    b. Enables client to participate in determining health care needs
    c. Uses such statements as "There is a new immunization available for meningitis caused by the hemophilus bacteria."
11. Encouraging client to make comparisons
    a. Helps clarify client's perception of a symptom
    b. Makes client aware of relationship between systems or events
    c. Includes such questions as "How is the pain similar or dissimilar to the pain you had last month?"
12. Encouraging client to describe how he perceives an event or symptom
    a. Shows nurse why a client is anxious, concerned, or doubtful about health care
    b. Avoids misconceptions by the nurse
    c. Includes such questions as "What do you think about that plan?"
13. Stating observations
    a. Increases client's awareness of a situation
    b. Shows client other's reaction to what he says or does
    c. Includes such questions as "Are you aware that you rub your eye a lot?"
14. Summing up
    a. Takes place at end of each part of history
    b. Offers chance to emphasize important points
    c. Provides sense of closure at end of total health history

H. Noneffective interviewing techniques/blocks to communication
1. Changing the subject
   a. Prevents client from completing a thought
   b. Shifts focus of conversation
2. Giving advice or false reassurance
   a. Jeopardizes the trusting relationship
   b. Preempts responsibility for client's health status instead of encouraging client to solve problems
   c. Includes such statements as "That job's not worth the risk to your health; if I were you I'd quit right away."
3. Jumping to conclusions
   a. Can result in inaccurate judgment and decision-making by the nurse
   b. Destroys rapport between client and nurse
   c. Includes such statements as: Client, "I've smoked two packs of cigarettes a day for 10 years." Nurse, "I'm sure you want to quit smoking. I can help you join a support group."
4. Asking leading or biased questions
   a. Suggests the "right" answer in the phrasing of the question
   b. Forces the client to give an "acceptable" response instead of an accurate one
   c. Includes such questions as "You have never had a venereal disease, have you?"
5. Repeating a question inappropriately
   a. Strikes client as preaching or nagging
   b. Annoys the client
   c. Includes such scenarios as: Nurse, "Have you reduced your cholesterol intake?" Client, "Yes, I avoid beef, pork, butter, and eggs." Nurse, "You know, high cholesterol foods aren't good for your heart."
6. Interfering with communication by recording health history in detail during interview; take notes instead

I. Documenting a subjective data base
1. Review data before final recording
2. Use pre-organized format to assist in recording
3. Be concise and specific
4. Label specific entries according to health history format
5. Avoid introductory phrases
6. Record data in client's own words
7. Record in detail all information relevant to each category
8. Use common abbreviations and symbols
9. Avoid use of "negative" or "normal" in descriptions
10. Date and sign health history; it is a legal document

J. Relationship between history (hx) and physical exam (PE)
1. History helps to focus physical exam
   a. Should be completed before PE
   b. Alerts examiner to existing or potential physical problems

      c. Establishes rapport between client and examiner
      d. Reveals previous experiences with health care system
      e. Presents client as whole person before the system by system exam
  2. Acts as a recall mechanism for current or future PE's
  3. Gives baseline data to others who later perform PE's or collect other objective data from client
  4. Safeguards against unnecessary trauma
      a. Allergies are known before performing lab or diagnostic procedures
      b. Painful or tender areas of body are known

K. Age and ethnic considerations
  1. Pediatric
      a. Include detailed perinatal history (prenatal, birth, neonatal)
      b. Include detailed nutritional history, especially for infant
      c. Note developmental milestones reached
      d. Note behavior, discipline, and school performance
      e. Obtain as much history as possible from child and so indicate in history
      f. Identify informant for pediatric history
  2. Geriatric
      a. Genetic history needs less emphasis; these problems are usually diagnosed at earlier age
      b. Elderly clients complain of pain less often than younger clients do
      c. Sensory losses, such as hearing loss, may make history taking more difficult
      d. Pharmaceutical history should be detailed
      e. Memory disorder or confusion may impede interview; use family or friends to validate history
      f. Isolated or lonely clients may be talkative; schedule more than one session
      g. Most geriatric clients have memory and intelligence intact; all should be treated with respect
  3. Ethnic
      a. Use interpreter if possible for clients who speak little English
      b. Be aware of differing cultural norms and values of people from other cultures; e.g., eye contact or expression of emotions may not be culturally acceptable
      c. It may be unacceptable to ask about certain parts of personal history, such as marital relationship or sexuality

L. Major techniques for collecting objective data
  1. Use of senses
      a. Sight
      b. Touch
      c. Smell
      d. Taste
      e. Hearing

2. Inspection: critically observing or visualizing client
    a. Observe client as total person
    b. Observe specific data for each system
    c. Observe behavior and body language
3. Palpation: using fingertips or palms to examine body parts
    a. Light palpation uses pads of fingers
    b. Deep palpation uses palmar surfaces and fingertips to detect position, size, shape, and mobility of a body part
    c. Sensing temperature uses dorsum of hand
4. Percussion: striking, thumping, or tapping a surface to vibrate structures and produce sound waves
    a. Determines density of area or structure
    b. Locates organ, demarcates boundaries
    c. Determines size and contour of underlying structure
    d. Uses middle finger of one hand on body surface as pleximeter and finger of other hand as plexor to strike a sharp blow to distal phalanx of pleximeter
    e. Assess loudness or intensity of percussion note
    f. Note pitch, duration, and quality
    g. Describe sound; for example, flat, dull
5. Auscultation: listening for sounds produced by human body, usually through a stethoscope
    a. Use over viscera
    b. Use over blood vessels
    c. Listen for same characteristics of sound described with percussion

M. Preparing client for objective data collection
1. Outline sequence of examination to reduce anxiety
2. Make certain client is warm and comfortable
3. Provide sufficient draping and an exam gown
4. Explain screening procedures
5. Summarize pertinent data from review of systems with client to identify problems and symptoms and focus on them
6. Convey warmth and relaxation
7. Establish rapport with client during history-taking prior to PE
8. If abnormality is detected during PE, question client about any related symptoms; explaining the examiner's findings at conclusion of exam reduces client anxiety
    a. Tell client his/her blood pressure
    b. Tell client results of screenings
    c. Inform client about heart and lung sounds
9. Proceed in head-to-toe fashion whenever possible

N. Major components of PE
1. General appearance and data from observation
2. Head and neck

3. Eyes
4. Ears
5. Nose, sinuses, mouth, and throat
6. Chest and respiratory system
7. Cardiovascular system
8. Breast
9. Abdomen
10. Genitourinary system
11. Musculoskeletal system
12. Neurologic system
13. Integument

O. Overview of laboratory and developmental screening procedures
1. Purposes of screening
    a. Used for case finding
    b. Not used for diagnosis
    c. Rescreen before referral if first screening abnormal
    d. Can be used on large numbers of people, such as at health fairs
2. Urinalysis screening
    a. Dipstick method
    b. Urine specific gravity
3. Blood glucose screening: dipstick with glucometer
4. Nutritional screening procedures
    a. Microhematocrit
    b. Height
    c. Weight
    d. Anthropometry
5. Hemoccult blood in feces
6. T.B. skin test
7. Infants and children screening procedures
    a. Developmental
    b. Speech
    c. Hearing
    d. Vision
8. Adult screening procedures
    a. Health risk appraisal
    b. Life stress inventory
    c. Vision
    d. Hearing
    e. Tonometry
9. Miscellaneous screening procedures; dependent on specific symptoms or problems
    a. Strep screening
    b. Pregnancy screening
    c. Substance abuse inventories

10. Screening exams requiring client education
    a. Rubella titer
    b. Cholesterol and triglycerides
    c. Venereal diseases
    d. Mammography

P. Recording objective data
1. Achieve a balance between conciseness and comprehensiveness
2. Describe findings; e.g., color, position, absence of lesions
3. Avoid use of "normal"
    a. Labeling fails to indicate what components were assessed
    b. Parameters of normal vary from client to client
4. Avoid use of subjective terms such as good, poor, or others
5. Be brief by using head-to-toe outline
    a. Sacrifice grammar
    b. Use phrases
    c. Use accepted abbreviations
6. Use sample recorded PE; especially helpful to inexperienced examiner
7. Examples of usually recorded parameters
    a. Movement
    b. Color
    c. Location
    d. Texture
    e. Contour
    f. Symmetry
    g. Size
8. Examples of descriptions of selected systems
    a. Head: normocephalic, no tenderness
    b. Cornea: clear; arcus senilis, right eye
    c. Cardiac: no pulsations, heaves, or lifts with inspection. PMI in 5th ICS. S_1 heard over mitral area. S_2 over pulmonic area. Rate 60 rhythm regular. No murmurs heard.

Q. Age and ethnic considerations in collection of objective data
1. Pediatrics
    a. Match PE to child's developmental level
    b. Do not proceed in head-to-toe fashion with infants and young children
    c. Examine ears and throat last
    d. Use distracting techniques for each age level; e.g., pacifier, puppets
    e. Examine infants and young children on parent's lap to facilitate cooperation
    f. Add or delete parts of PE depending on age, such as head circumference, scoliosis screening
    g. Be aware of age-related differences in PE findings; e.g., vital signs
    h. Include specific developmental screening tests in any exam of infants and young children; e.g., Denver Developmental Screening Test (DDST)

2. Geriatrics
   a. Allow more time for PE
   b. May need to adjust positioning; e.g., for pelvic exam
   c. Be aware of the specific screening exams required for this age group; e.g., tonometry and colonic cancer screening
3. Ethnic considerations
   a. Women from Eastern cultures, e.g., Moslems, Chinese, have rigid beliefs about modesty. Examiner must instruct carefully and alter exam to accommodate beliefs
   b. Examiner must be aware of cultural values related to childrearing when performing P.E. on children
   c. Special screening procedures are done for persons in certain ethnic groups; e.g., sickle cell screening for Blacks

P- what provokes it - what doing
relives it

Q quality - dull ache sharp

R- Region - Radiation
Show where it is.
does it spread.

S - severidity
Scale 1-10 (worst)
did you stop what you were doing

T- timing - start
constant
comes and goes.

Past medical

Points to Remember

Health assessment is based on a theoretical framework that includes principles from systems theory, developmental theories, and psychosocial theories.

The health assessment relies on a subjective data base (health history) and an objective data base (physical examination, screening methods).

Nursing diagnoses are derived from an analysis of both data bases.

The subjective data base prepares a focus for the physical exam and establishes rapport with the client.

Techniques for physical examination include: use of senses, inspection, percussion, palpation, and auscultation.

Age and ethnic considerations are necessary parts of the health assessment process.

Glossary

Congruent communication—communication in which verbal and non-verbal messages are consistent

Ethnicity—the cultural and social characteristics of a group of people

Nonverbal communication—facial expressions, eye contact, and movements of extremities that provide information about emotions

Objective data—information that is verifiable through direct observation, laboratory tests, screening procedures, or physical examination

Psychosocial considerations—influences on behavior that grow out of the interaction between an individual and his social environment, as mediated by human system, social systems, economic systems, cultural systems, and the physical environment

Subjective data—information the client gives to the health care provider about his/her health status. Subjective data can also be obtained from a client's family or friends

Current Health Status

Learning Objectives

After studying this section, the reader should be able to:

• List the biographical data needed for a complete health assessment.

• Understand why it is essential to know the client's reason for seeking health care.

• Perform a complete history of present illness (HPI), including symptom analysis.

• List the elements of health promotion and protection.

• Make an objective assessment of a client's health-promoting and protecting behaviors.

II. Current Health Status

A. Biographic/demographical information: data that identify client and provide clues to his/her epidemiologic risks
1. Name
    a. First/middle/last/married woman's maiden name
    b. Name that client wishes to use
    c. Last name of spouse or parent if different from client
2. Address
    a. Current home address
    b. Current mailing address (if different from home address)
    c. Permanent address where client can always be reached (if different from home address)
3. Telephone number
    a. Current home phone
    b. Current work phone
    c. If no phone, number where client can be reached
4. Social security number
5. Sex
6. Current age in years (months if less than 2 years)
7. Date of birth: month/day/year
8. Place of birth
9. Race
10. Nationality/culture/ethnic group
11. Religion
12. Marital status
13. Household members
14. Education level
15. Occupation
16. Historian (client or other)
    a. Caregiver's assessment of historian reliability
    b. If other, relationship to and knowledge of client

B. Current health status: the client's perception of present health and how this may differ from usual health status
1. Reason for visit: "Why are you here today?" (See Part C)
    a. If the reason is illness-related, it is known as the chief complaint
    b. Always record the reason in the client's own words; paraphrasing may change meaning
2. History of present illness (HPI) if appropriate
    a. What does client think illness is, and why
    b. When did it begin
    c. How long has it lasted
    d. Describe its course
    e. What are its signs and symptoms (for each major symptom, do a symptom analysis; see Part D); in what order did they develop

    f. What remedies/medications/treatments has client tried; what works and what doesn't

    g. How have symptoms changed; how is the illness currently bothering the client; is it getting better/worse

    h. What effect has the illness had on client's life

    i. What does client think caused illness

    j. Does client know others with similar symptoms

    k. Has client had a similar illness before

    l. How is client and client's family coping

3. Other known health problems
4. Health concerns or worries
5. Health needs; areas for improvement
6. When did client last feel healthy
7. What changes motivated this visit
8. Which issues does client want to discuss today

C. Reason for seeking health care, and what client hopes to accomplish by seeking care

1. The stated reason for seeking care may not be the actual reason for seeking care
2. Common reasons
   a. Periodic health assessment for preventive health care
   b. Examination required for school or job
   c. Examination motivated by non-specific anxieties or symptoms of aging
   d. Referral from another caregiver agency
   e. A return appointment following a prior visit
   f. Minor acute symptoms not responding to self-care
   g. Subacute symptom(s) which have become chronic
   h. Subacute symptom(s) with implications for major problems
   i. Psychological/mental health distress
   j. Desire for advice/help with lifestyle change
   k. Major, acute symptom(s)
3. Client expectation from visit
   a. Based on prior experience with health care system
   b. Based on personal and social considerations: locus of control, age, support system, cultural definition of health/illness
   c. Based on usual health status
   d. Based on the real reason for seeking care; e.g., if seeking lifestyle change, client may expect to learn about alternative health habits; if client has mental health problems, he/she may expect understanding, reassurance, or referral
4. Importance/implications of knowing the client's reason for seeking health care
   a. The real reason will determine the client's expectations for outcome
   b. The client's physical and psychological condition influences the degree of assessment that can be tolerated

     c. Both client and caregiver must verbalize their expectations of the course and desired outcome of the visit

     d. The client must understand the limitations of what the caregiver can do

D. Symptom analysis: the systematic process of collecting a subjective data base about the client's major complaint(s). Component parts include:

1. Location: where in the body does the symptom reside; be specific

PQRST 2. Quality: the acuity, degree, and sensation of symptoms; how they interfere with lifestyle or relationships

3. Quantity: the severity, intensity, frequency, size of symptoms

4. Temporal characteristics: symptom onset, duration, periodicity

5. Setting: where and under what circumstances the symptom appears

6. Aggravating factors: what makes the symptom worse; e.g., environmental factors

7. Alleviating factors: what makes the symptom better

8. Associated manifestations: related and potentially related symptoms

E. Health protection and promotion behaviors

1. Purposes in collecting this data
   a. Personal health habits affect overall health. A health history is incomplete without this data
   b. The client's level of participation in promoting own health affects the client/caregiver relationship and the way health information and education is provided
   c. The client's expectation of the health assessment is determined by perception of client/caregiver roles. Caregiver needs to understand the client's health locus of control to make an encounter effective

2. Pattern of health care
   a. Circumstances under which client seeks professional health care
   b. Persons/occupations to whom client goes for health care
   c. Client's description of what he/she does to stay healthy
   d. Exams/screenings periodically sought and date of last exam

3. Locus of control/self care
   a. Locus of control: individual's perception of whether control over his health is internal or external
   b. Self-care: activities initiated and performed by the individual to maintain life, health, and well-being. What is client's philosophy and practice of self-care in health promotion, health maintenance, specific disease prevention, diagnosis and treatment of symptoms, decision to seek professional health care
   c. Learning style: by determining how a client learns, the nurse can tailor health education; a visual learner learns by watching a demonstration, an auditory learner learns by listening, an experiential learner learns by doing, an intellectual learner learns by reading

4. Risk factor analysis: an estimation of personal risk for mortality from specified conditions; various tools to measure risk are available
   a. Based on actuarial data; requires a prepared program
   b. Based on family health history, personal health history, present health status, and health habits
   c. Affected by synergistic effects; the risk involved in having three factors may exceed the sum of having each one
   d. Can show how risk of illness decreases in response to specified life style changes, such as weight loss
   e. Commonly collected data may include weight, diet, blood cholesterol, smoking level, family history of heart disease/stroke, seat belt use, alcohol consumption, exercise level
   f. Includes such conditions as heart disease, cancer, stroke, motor vehicle accidental death, cirrhosis, arteriosclerosis
5. Client's self-concept and coping patterns
   a. Feelings about his/her physical capabilities as compared to peers
   b. Feelings about his/her cognitive abilities as compared to peers
   c. Satisfaction with his/her relationships with family and friends as compared to peers
   d. Satisfaction with self at this time
   e. Satisfaction with his/her current age; if dissatisfied, ask what age would be better and why
   f. Feelings about his/her emotional stability and about the ways in which emotions can be recognized and expressed
   g. Feelings about his/her problem-solving ability and methods used
   h. Feelings about ability to handle stress: how to express it, its health effects, how it was handled in the past, what coping methods work best, who helps
   i. Experiences with problems or stresses client cannot cope with
6. Relaxation/stress reduction
   a. Degree to which this is important to client
   b. Degree to which client needs this
   c. Potential stress-reduction methods: meditation, strenuous physical activity, guided imagery, diversional activity, biofeedback, massage, hydrotherapy, artistic pursuit (music, dance, pottery), etc.
   d. Current choice and level of purposeful relaxation; adequacy of time and method, desired level of use
7. Exercise
   a. Its importance to client
   b. Extent of client's desire to change in this area
   c. Client's goal in exercise/fitness: cardiovascular fitness, muscular endurance, musculoskeletal flexibility, musculoskeletal coordination, muscular strength, general feeling of well-being
   d. Present type of exercise and level of activity
   e. Knowledge and use of proper warm up, cool down, and body mechanics
   f. Types of exercise client enjoys

8. Nutrition
   a. Client's perception of nutrition's effect on health
   b. Value client accords to nutritional self-care
   c. Client's rating of current nutritional adequacy
   d. Client's perception of current weight compared to ideal weight
   e. Client's food preferences; allergies/special dietary needs
   f. How client would like to change current diet
   g. 24-hour recall: list of everything consumed during last 24 hours, by amount; compare this with Recommended Daily Allowances to provide basis for nutritional counseling
   h. Client's consumption pattern: three meals versus skips breakfast, etc.
   i. Client's control over dietary change: who plans meals, cooks, etc.
   j. Use of nutritional supplements
9. Dental self-care
   a. Its importance to client
   b. Extent of client's desire to work/improve
   c. Current self-care habits: frequency and quality of brushing/flossing, use of other mechanical aids (Waterpik, toothpick, etc.), type of brush used, type of toothpaste used, history of fluoride use
   d. Frequency of seeking professional dental care
10. Substance use
   a. Tobacco: history of use, type of use, amount of use, desire to quit
   b. Alcohol: history of use; amount and pattern of use per week; did client ever feel a need to cut down, or feel guilty about drinking; was client ever annoyed by criticism about his/her drinking; does he/she wish to change drinking habits
   c. Medications; regular use of prescription and nonprescription medicine (what and for what purposes), pattern of use, concern about amount of use, desire to change current practice
   d. Street drugs: current use, pattern of use, kinds used, desire to change current practice, concerns about use, history of past use
11. Seat belt use
   a. Its importance to client
   b. Extent of client's felt need for improvement
   c. Assessment of current use
   d. Client's belief in effectiveness of seat belt use
   e. Client's goal regarding seat belt use

Points to Remember

Biographical data makes possible precise client identification and provides initial clues to client's potential health risks.

The actual reason for the client's visit determines his expectation of the visit course and outcome.

A client's health locus of control, philosophy of self-care, and learning style indicate the best way to approach client and optimize health learning.

Personal lifestyle and health habits are the most important predictors of health and longevity; health habits significantly influence a person's risk of premature mortality.

Taking a history is also an opportunity for health education.

Glossary

Demographic—pertaining to statistics about a given population; for example, births, deaths

Locus of control—a person's perception of whether control over the course of his/ her own life and health is internal or external

Risk—the probability of incurring a disease or condition

Signs and symptoms—Signs are objective evidence of illness or abnormality; symptoms are subjective evidence perceived by client

Stress—non-specific physiologic responses to actual, potential, or imagined demands placed on client

Health History: Physical, Family, and Social

Learning Objectives

After studying this section, the reader should be able to:

• Identify major components of past health, family, and personal social history.

• Develop a genogram for family history.

• Understand and communicate to client the relationship of each assessment area to his overall health.

• Describe age and ethnic considerations in obtaining health history.

• Record subjective data from health history, family history, and personal social history.

III. Health History: Physical, Family, and Social

A. Physical health history
1. Purposes
   a. Identifies all major health problems of client
   b. Provides information; assists with management of present problems
   c. Links data about current problem with past health problems
   d. Identifies client's methods for preventing illness
2. Birth and physical development history
   a. Significant events
   b. Complications, treatments, sequelae
3. Childhood illnesses
   a. Rubella, rubeola, mumps, pertussis
   b. Chickenpox, other rash illnesses
   c. Strep throat, scarlet fever, rheumatic fever
   d. Frequent ear infections, pneumonia, bronchitis
   e. Age of onset, course, complications of each illness
   f. Frequency of physician visits
4. Immunizations
   a. Date of last tetanus shot
   b. Childhood immunization hx (DPT, OPV, MMR)
   c. Immunizations for travel
   d. Others (influenza, HiB, pneumonia)
   e. Immunoglobulin
5. Allergies
   a. Drug allergens: types of reaction and name of drug(s)
   b. Environmental agents or irritants
   c. Food allergens: types of foods and description of reaction
   d. Animals (including insects): animal names and reactions
   e. Allergy prevention
   f. Allergy treatment
   g. History of anaphylactic reaction
6. Hospitalization for surgery or serious illness
   a. Date(s)
   b. Reason
   c. Duration of hospitalization
   d. Surgical procedures and/or medical treatments
   e. Complications
   f. Course of recovery
   g. Type of follow-up care
   h. Sequelae
   i. Continued medication and/or treatment
7. Illnesses not requiring hospitalization
   a. Status of chronic illnesses such as diabetes, T.B.
   b. Serious infectious disease; hepatitis, mononucleosis
   c. Frequent colds, sore throat

        d. Unexplained fever
        e. Complications
        f. Use of prescription medication
        g. Use of home remedies or over-the-counter drugs

8. Accidents and injuries
        a. Broken bones, dislocations
        b. Head injury with loss of consciousness
        c. Other types of injury; e.g., poisoning
        d. Causes of and treatments for injuries
        e. Complications, sequelae

9. Obstetrical history
        a. Number of pregnancies, planned or unplanned
        b. Miscarriages, therapeutic abortions
        c. Prenatal care
        d. Course of pregnancy, labor, delivery
        e. Live births
        f. Dates of births
        g. Maternal age at births
        h. Perinatal complications
        i. Postpartum illness

B. Family history

1. Purposes
        a. To learn about hereditary or communicable disorders that might affect client's health status
        b. To learn about health status of client's blood relatives, including maternal and paternal grandparents, parents, siblings, children, uncles and aunts
        c. To learn about health status of immediate family members
        d. To identify environmental factors in a family system that could affect client's health status
        e. To educate clients about genetic disorders and refer them for counseling

2. Major disorders to inquire about
        a. Heart disease
        b. Hypertension, stroke
        c. Cancer
        d. Mental retardation
        e. Hematologic disorders; e.g., hemophilia, sickle cell anemia
        f. Diabetes
        g. Epilepsy
        h. Allergic disorders; e.g., asthma
        i. Tuberculosis
        j. Obesity
        k. Kidney disease
        l. Mental illness; e.g., manic-depression
        m. Arthritis
        n. Known genetic disorders such as cystic fibrosis or Huntington's chorea

3. Additional necessary information
   a. Age and state of health of living grandparents, parents, siblings, children, aunts and uncles
   b. Deceased family members, age at death
   c. Cause of death
   d. Severe health problems of living relatives
4. Family tree diagram or genogram provides clear visual representation of family health history and impact on client health (See figure below)

Sample genogram

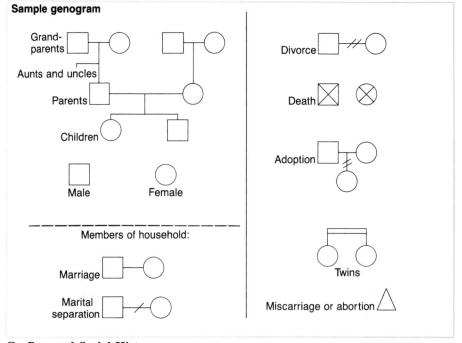

C. Personal Social History

1. Purposes
   a. Assess psychosocial aspects of past and present life
   b. Assess impact of psychosocial influences on health
   c. Assess quality of life based on psychosocial factors
2. Environmental assessment: encompasses one's living space, neighborhood, and community; all contain hazards affecting physical health, risk of injury, mental health, and family health
   a. Living space: adequacy of total space, availability of privacy, adequacy of light and heat, noise level, safety hazards, pollutants/allergens in air and water
   b. Neighborhood: safety of neighborhood, adequacy of lighting, adequacy and safety of play areas/streets/sidewalks/yards/transportation, availability

of police/fire/ambulance, availability of garbage service, availability of services for groceries/drugs/health, lack of hazards (open dumpsters, litter, rats, etc.)

c. Community: purity of air and water, adequate open space, adequate emergency and health care services, availability of resources to help meet health/social/economic needs, client knowledge of resources appropriate to his/her needs, effects of weather and climate

3. Assessment of cultural/religious background and practices: significant influences on values, beliefs, family life, definition of health and illness, and personal philosophy

   a. Client's culture/race/religion may result in a different lifestyle/belief system than others in the community

   b. Client's cultural/ethnic/religious history: general history of group up to present generation, client's physical closeness to culture, client's moral or spiritual closeness with identified group; how beliefs and values of identified group differ from other groups

   c. Client's global orientations: man-nature orientation (role of man in the broader environment; harmony versus mastery), life-death orientation (the meaning and acceptance of the latter relative to the former), power and status orientation (social mobility versus rigidity; acceptance of place in society), time orientation (meaning of past, present, future; adherence to clock time), distance orientation (degree of physical closeness to another person allowed in different contexts)

   d. Description of social structures in group: religion and its importance, educational system, kinship system, political system, economic system, social stratification, important social institutions

   e. Home: who lives in home, spatial relationships of home, concept of territory, concept of property, sleeping arrangements

   f. Family: who is considered part of family, roles of family members

   g. Health and illness: definition of health and illness; at what point client is sick; causes of illness; what restores health, how types of ill health are differentiated, how mental illness is defined and viewed; common health problems, common problems that are uncommon in client's experience; nutritional practices, including everyday diet pattern and dietary changes associated with illness; views about sexually-related functions

   h. Health care system roles: caring practices (who cares for infants, children, women during pregnancy/abortion/delivery, new mothers, ill persons, the infirm, aged, dying); caregivers' preparation, functions, societal status, levels of practice, levels of treatment; health problems experienced by client or family member because of cultural background

4. Assessment of family and social support systems: people to whom client feels closest; they have the most influence on socialization, lifestyle, values, self-concept, health behaviors, and compliance with health regimens

   a. Family system relationships: who is identified as family, who is the most important family member(s) in client's life; importance of family in client's present life; who makes major decisions affecting client; family ability and methods of coping with stress; family ability and methods of dealing with conflict; client satisfaction with family support/acceptance/ help with problem solving; satisfaction with family love/affection; satisfaction with shared family time; perception of his/her roles in family; recent major changes or foreseeable changes

b. Other social support systems: who are identified as support systems, who is identified as the most significant person(s), importance of these persons/groups in client's life; client satisfaction with support systems' help with problem-solving/acceptance/support; satisfaction with support systems' love/affection; satisfaction with time spent with support persons; client's perception of his/her roles in support systems; recent major changes or foreseeable changes

5. Assessment of socioeconomic status: informal societal stratification based on upbringing, education, occupation, and/or income. The most common denominators are:

a. Social class: based mainly on occupation as the primary indicator of prestige; probably the prime influence on a family's lifestyle. The best classification of family social class is still the this one: upper classes (upper-upper, the established wealthy families and lower-upper, the newly wealthy), middle classes (upper-middle, the solid business and professional group, often the civic leaders, and lower-middle, the small business people, white-collar workers, and some skilled tradespeople), lower classes (upper-lower, the blue-collar workers and lower-lower, the unskilled or unemployed, poverty-level families)

b. Economic level: can be estimated by social class and occupation; since there may be confounding factors, such as level of outstanding debt or a member's health care expenses, a separate assessment needs to be made based on the following information: major sources of family income, major outstanding debts or unusual ongoing expenses, adequacy of income for living expenses, adequacy of income for recreation, vacation, extras, extent of current health insurance, availability of savings, degree of worry about family finances

6. Occupational/educational history: educational preparation, work history, and occupational satisfaction are important because of their relationship to mental health, self-concept, socioeconomic status, safety factors, and environmental hazards

a. Current primary occupation (including homemaking or student)
b. Length of time in that role
c. Other concurrent occupations
d. Satisfaction with current work role(s)
e. Degree of stress in current work role(s)
f. Highest educational level achieved and major area(s) of study; educational goal
g. Satisfaction in student role (past and present)
h. Occupational history, occupational goal
i. Safety/environmental risks identified in work setting(s); ways in which client attempts to minimize risk(s)

7. Assessment of behavioral styles: environmental modifications of temperament; temperamental styles are identifiable very early in life, but continue to act on, and be acted on by, other areas of the client's life
   a. Quick-tempered versus even-tempered
   b. Moody versus easy-going
   c. Trusting versus suspicious
   d. Calm versus excitable
   e. Relaxed versus tense
   f. Quick moving/speaking versus slow moving/speaking
   g. Avoidance of new experiences versus enthusiasm for new experiences
   h. Predictable behavior versus unpredictable behavior
   i. Assertive/leading versus passive/following
   j. Adaptable versus rigid
   k. Happy/cheerful versus sad/gloomy
   l. Extroverted versus introverted
8. Sexuality and reproduction patterns: knowledge, feelings, and satisfaction with the sexual part of life; has implications for physical, emotional, family, and social health
   a. Whether client is sexually active, and client's sexual orientation/ satisfaction with current level of sexual activity
   b. Satisfaction with current knowledge about sex
   c. Preparation for puberty, feelings about early sexual adjustment
   d. Past/current contraceptive practice, satisfaction with method
   e. Reproductive history: success in conceiving children, satisfaction with pregnancy and childbirth (mother and father), number of living and non-living children, satisfaction with parental role, desire for children or more children
   f. Knowledge and feelings about menopause, if applicable
   g. Way(s) in which sex/sexuality may negatively affect other areas of health or satisfaction
9. Assessment of recent life changes/stressors: a significant and predictable relationship exists between the number or magnitude of stressful life events and the onset and seriousness of physical illness. Assessing recent life stressors both as a predictor and to assist in prevention of disease is critical
10. Assessment of biological rhythms: patterns differ from individual to individual; variance from normal rhythms can be a cause or an effect of sub-optimal health
    a. Daily energy pattern: "day" or "night" person; best and worst times of day; fit of present daily routine with inner rhythm, satisfaction with routine, impact on well-being when routine changes
    b. Scheduling of time: personal preference for having time scheduled or unscheduled, satisfaction with current amount of scheduling in life, satisfaction with amount of control over current schedule and routine

    c. Sleep/wake rhythm: number of hours of sleep needed to feel good, number of hours of sleep presently averaged per day, frequency of wakefulness during sleep cycle, regularity of dreaming, content and recurrence of similar dreams, tendency of dreams to frighten or awaken client

    d. Hunger pattern: times of day client feels hungry, fit of hunger rhythm with meal pattern both in timing and size, effect of inability to follow rhythm

    e. Elimination rhythm: client's perception of patterning of urge to void and/or move bowels, ability to respond to urges without stress, effect of inability to follow pattern

11. Description of typical day: focus on the variety, timing, and feelings about daily routines/events; helps identify stressors, relationships, life satisfaction, and ability to perform activities of daily living (ADL)

    a. Detailed description of a normal day from waking up to falling asleep. Have client use yesterday as the example if it was typical. Examiner should note: body language during description, affect, verbal descriptions used; note pace of day, availability of private time and space, availability of relaxation, support systems contacted, feelings at the beginning and end of the day, amount of satisfaction versus frustration expressed

    b. Impact of current health problems on daily routines

    c. Ability to perform the ADL necessary to meet needs for rest, nutrition, elimination, hygiene, ambulation/transportation, communication, and performance of family/home roles

12. Recreational activities: assess the degree to which a client finds diversion, relaxation, and/or meets personal goals apart from work and family obligations

    a. Perceived value of recreation to client

    b. Leisure time identified and planned for by the client; who plans the activities and who participates

    c. Recreational activities pursued: sports, hobbies, passive listening/watching, relaxation activity, or civic/cultural/educational pursuits

    d. Time spent on recreation versus time client would like to spend

    e. Satisfaction gained from each activity

    f. Persons with whom client chooses to spend recreational time

13. Psychosocial developmental assessment: nursing uses broad developmental models as a base for assessing psychosocial health status and needs. Different nursing curricula, practices, and/or individual nurses may view clients from a variety of developmental theories; assessments will depend on the specific developmental framework within which the client is studied. Following is a list of theories often used by nurses:

    a. Eric Erikson: described psychosocial development within eight epigenetic life cycle stages, each of which requires the completion of specified developmental tasks. Positive and negative outcomes of the stages have been identified and may be assessed

  b. Sigmund Freud: described psychosexual development as the major force in the development of personality and emotional organization. The major influence on Erikson

  c. Arnold Gesell: described development as the combination of biological, cultural, and familial influences with the latter mediating between the others

  d. Lawrence Kohlberg: described moral development as a process similar to Erikson's; children develop, through identification and positive reinforcement, a personal value system and sense of morality that is greatly influenced by the family

  e. Jean Piaget: described cognitive development as the result of central nervous system maturation interacting with a culture and its educational process

  f. Developmental theories of aging: specific to the period of aging, these range from the continuity theory of Neugarten (basic behavior patterns continue through the aging process), to the activity theory of Havighurst (the behaviors/tasks of middle age should continue throughout the rest of life), to the disengagement theory of Cumming and Henry (the aging individual and society gradually disengage from each other, making death a more mutually satisfactory end for both)

  g. Family development: Evelyn Duvall divided the family life cycle into eight stages, basing them primarily on the age of the oldest child and assigning developmental tasks to each stage

D. Age and ethnic considerations

 1. Pediatric

  a. Health of mother during pregnancy with client

  b. History of labor and delivery

  c. History of nursery stay

  d. Neonatal history

 2. Geriatric

  a. Hereditary diseases need less attention since they are usually identified at an earlier age

  b. Childhood illnesses may be difficult to recall

  c. Past health history may be long and complex: childhood illnesses may have been more complex prior to antibiotics and immunizations

 3. Ethnic

  a. General information: be aware of each ethnic group's specific genetic disorders. Realize that people from other cultures may be reluctant to discuss folk medicine unless interviewer indicates interest and acceptance of those practices

  b. Blacks: sickle-cell anemia, hypertension

  c. Persons of Mediterranean descent: thalassemia

  d. Persons of Jewish descent: Tay-Sachs disease

  e. Anglos/Middle European: cystic fibrosis, muscular dystrophy

Points to Remember

Areas to cover under a past health history include illnesses, hospitalizations, surgery, allergies, accidents and immunizations.

Family history focuses on inherited familial or environmental diseases in blood relatives and spouses.

A genogram is a diagram of the family history.

A more detailed perinatal health history is needed for children.

Ethnic and racial groups have genetic disorders specific to the group.

Glossary

Biological rhythms—physiologic processes recurring at regular intervals

Cystic fibrosis, sickle cell anemia, Tay-Sachs disease, and thalassemia—autosomal recessive disorders specific to particular racial groups

Genogram—a schematic representation of family history

Stressor—a physical or psychological force that disrupts the equilibrium of or produces strain in a structure, system, or organism; a cause of stress

Review of Systems

Learning Objectives
After studying this section, the reader should be able to:

- Understand the purposes of a systematic review:
  —for the client
  —for the examiner.

- List the data to be collected when reviewing each area of the body.

- Identify the anatomic/physiologic system to which each datum relates.

- Relate age- and ethnic-appropriate variations in the review.

IV. Review of Systems

A. Definition: systematic collection of subjective data about the parts and systems of the body

B. Purposes of systematic review
1. For the client
   a. Helps the client remember pertinent information by grouping related data
   b. Helps the client understand relationships between data by asking about each system separately
2. For the examiner
   a. Provides a checklist to validate and organize subjective data
   b. Helps the examiner form impressions about the client's health status
   c. Provides focus for the physical assessment by identifying systems with potential health problems/concerns

C. Data to be gathered about each part or system of the body
1. General
   a. Current/usual state of health
   b. Ability to carry out ADL
   c. Exercise patterns and tolerance
   d. Frequency of illness
   e. Recent weight change, fatigue, weakness, fever, sweating
2. Head and neck
   a. Headache: type, site, frequency, duration, cause, remedies
   b. History (hx) of head trauma, loss of consciousness
   c. Dizziness, vertigo, syncope
   d. Scalp: itching, lesions, infestations, scaling
   e. Hair: color, distribution, texture, amount, alopecia
   f. Face: significant scars, lesions, nevi; hair distribution
   g. Neck: pain, stiffness, limited range of motion (ROM), swelling, masses
   h. Hx of infection, disease, surgery, treatment, medication
3. Eyes
   a. Vision problems, recent changes, use of corrective lenses, last vision exam, glaucoma exam, cataracts, color blindness
   b. Diplopia, blurred vision, blind areas, decrease in visual field, halo around visual fields, spots in front of eyes
   c. Eye pain, itching, excessive tearing, light sensitivity, discharge
   d. Eyelid swelling, styes, tics
   e. Hx of trauma, disease, surgery, treatment, medication
4. Ears
   a. Hearing problems, recent changes, use of hearing aid, last hearing exam, noise exposure
   b. Ringing in ears, unexplained noises, sensitivity to certain noises
   c. Ear pain, itching, drainage, cerumen characteristics
   d. Dizziness, vertigo

    e. Hx of frequent infections, ruptured eardrums, mastoiditis, disease, surgery, treatment, medication

5. Nose and paranasal sinuses
   a. Sense of smell, recent changes
   b. Inflammation, discharge, nose bleed, obstruction
   c. Postnasal drip, sinus pain
   d. Frequent sneezing, watery drainage, allergic reactions
   e. Mouth breathing, snoring
   f. Hx of frequent infection, allergy, trauma, disease, surgery, treatment, medication

6. Mouth and throat
   a. Cracked lips, dry lips, cold sores, lesions on lips
   b. Taste sensations, recent changes
   c. Bleeding, swelling, pain, lesions, receding gums; buccal surface lesions
   d. Tongue coated, cracked, with soreness, lesions
   e. Teeth: completeness, condition, hygiene, use of dentures, last dental exam, pain
   f. Difficulty chewing or swallowing; grinds teeth
   g. Hoarseness, recent voice change
   h. Sore throat, enlarged or absent tonsils
   i. Hx of frequent throat infections, disease, surgery, treatment, medication

7. Cardiovascular (CV)
   a. Chest pain, palpitations, shortness of breath (on exertion, at rest, or reclining), uneven heart rate
   b. Recent changes, last CV exam, last EKG, last blood pressure
   c. Hx of murmur, disease, hypertension, surgery, treatment, medication
   d. Peripheral vascular: edema, cyanosis, pallor, coldness, numbness, varicosities, intermittent cramping in extremities; hx of phlebitis

8. Respiratory/Thoracic
   a. Shortness of breath (SOB), painful breathing, wheezing
   b. Cough, sputum production, blood in sputum, sweating at night
   c. Smoking habits
   d. Recent changes, last respiratory exam, last chest X-ray, last TB test
   e. Hx of infection, disease, lesion, surgery, treatment, medication
   f. Thoracic trauma, pain, tenderness

9. Breast
   a. Pain, tenderness, lumps, nipple discharge
   b. Breast enlargement in males
   c. Breast changes during menstrual cycle
   d. Recent changes, last professional breast exam, pattern of self-breast exam, date of last mammography
   e. Axillary tenderness, masses
   f. Hx of infection, disease, surgery, treatment, medication
   g. Breast feeding history in females

10. Gastrointestinal (GI)
    a. Nausea, vomiting, indigestion, belching, pain related to eating

    b. Food intolerances, appetite change

    c. Jaundice, abdominal swelling or tenderness

    d. Diarrhea, constipation, flatulence, stool characteristics, bowel habits

    e. Rectal pain, hemorrhoids, rectal bleeding

    f. Recent changes, last GI examination

    g. Hx of infection, disease, surgery, treatment, medication

11. Genitourinary (GU)

    a. Urine characteristics: color, clarity, odor, presence of blood, pus, stones

    b. Urination characteristics: frequency, comfort, increased or decreased output, nocturia, difficulty starting stream, incontinence (with or without stress), change in stream

    c. Tenderness, lesions, masses, discharge, odor, itching, burning in genitourinary area

    d. Pain in flank area

    e. Tenderness, inflammation, lumps in groin

    f. Satisfaction with sexual adjustment, use of contraception, knowledge of safe sex practice, onset of puberty

    g. Hx of infection, disease, venereal disease, surgery, infertility, sterilization, treatment, medication

    Females only:

    h. Description of menstrual cycle, characteristics of menstrual period, date of last menstrual period

    i. Sanitary protection

    j. Obstetrical hx, complications

    k. Recent changes, date of last gynecologic exam, date and result of last Pap smear

    Males only:

    l. Foreskin present or absent

    m. Hx of hernia, hydrocele, date of last testicular exam, knowledge and practice of testicular self-exam

    n. Tenderness, enlargement, or inflammation of prostate, hx of disease, surgery, treatment

12. Musculoskeletal (MSK)

    a. Muscle weakness, atrophy, cramping, aching, spasm, tremors

    b. Joint stiffness, aching, swelling, deformity, limited movement, crepitation

    c. Handedness

    d. Gait stiff, uncoordinated, jerky

    e. Flat-footed, feet toe in or out

    f. Back stiffness, limited movement, deformity, poor posture

    g. Hx of trauma, fractures, dislocation, disease, surgery, treatment, medication

13. Endocrine

    a. Change in skin color, pattern of pigmentation, hair distribution and texture

    b. Heat/cold tolerance, excessive/absent sweating, unexplained growth, change in energy level, change in sexual vigor, exophthalmic

    c. Excessive hunger, thirst, urination

    d. Thyroid growth

    e. Recent changes, last test for sugar in blood or urine, last test for thyroid condition

    f. Hx of disease, treatment, medication, hormone therapy

14. Hematopoietic/Lymphatic

    a. Tendency to bleed or bruise easily

    b. Unexplained appearance of petechiae or ecchymoses

    c. Pallor, fatigue, appearance of dark circles around eyes

    d. Hx of disease, anemia, blood transfusion, treatment, medication

    e. Lymph node tenderness, swelling

15. Integument

    a. Skin color, texture, pigmentation, moisture

    b. Rash, lesions, wounds, itching

    c. Skin tumors, swelling, pain

    d. Hair texture, amount, distribution

    e. Nail characteristics: texture, thickness, brittleness, growth pattern, deformity, color, shape

    f. Recent changes

    g. Hx of trauma, infection, disease, surgery, treatment, medication

16. Immunologic

    a. Frequency of infection, secondary infection, rate of healing

    b. Frequency and timing of sneezing, watery nasal discharge, watery eyes

    c. Frequency and timing of airway disturbances

    d. Frequency and timing of skin eruptions, itching, hives

    e. Recent changes, date of last allergy testing

    f. Hx of disease, treatment, medication

17. Neurologic/Mental status

    a. Headache

    b. Anxiety, irritability, tremors, spasms, sleep disturbance, seizures, dizziness, loss of consciousness

    c. Disturbance of memory (short- or long-term), disorientation, confusion, mood shifts

    d. Difficulty in performance of social behaviors

    e. Sensory perceptual disturbances or changes in ability to see, hear, smell, taste, articulate

    f. Change in writing ability, comprehension of speech or written word

    g. Motor and coordination ability disturbances or changes in gait, posture, balance, bilaterally equal muscle strength, hand-eye coordination, performance of purposeful motor activity

    h. Sensory ability disturbances or changes in discrimination of touch/tickling/pain sensations, increased/decreased sensitivity to sensation anywhere

18. Other
    a. Additional symptoms not questioned about
    b. Other recent changes concerning client
    c. Which symptoms/conditions/changes are most significant to client

D. Age and ethnic appropriate variations or areas of particular significance
1. Pediatric (assuming a parent as historian)
    a. General: growth patterns
    b. Head and neck: closure of fontanel
    c. Eyes: visual acuity, squinting, head tilt when looking, inequality of gaze, rapid blinking
    d. Ears: hearing acuity (unilateral and bilateral), frequency of otitis media, history of myringotomy
    e. Nose and sinuses: frequency of epistaxis, rhinitis, mouth breathing
    f. Mouth and throat: pattern of dentition, fluoride use, dental hygiene, frequency of sore throat/tonsillitis, frequency of lesions in mouth
    g. CV: hx of murmur, SOB with exertion
    h. Respiratory: history of croup, asthma
    i. Breast: supernumerary nipples, age/sex related breast development
    j. GI: age of toilet training, elimination pattern, presence or hx of umbilical hernia, hx of rectal itch/pinworms
    k. GU: age of toilet training, frequency of bed wetting after fourth birthday, genital irritation/itching, masturbation, age-related sexual development
    l. Musculoskeletal (MSK): posture, spinal curvature, congenital defects/treatment, muscle cramps, joint stiffness/deformity/swelling, complaints of pain
    m. Endocrine: rapid or slow growth, precocious or delayed puberty, excessive hunger/thirst/urination, change in hair distribution
    n. Hematopoietic/lymphatic: pallor, fatigue, bleeding/bruising, frequent lymph node enlargement
    o. Integument: hx of rash diseases, frequency of skin problems, acne (onset/severity/treatment), infestations
    p. Immunologic/allergic: frequency and timing of infection/dermatitis/rhinitis/food intolerance/asthma, known allergies, allergy testing/treatment
    q. Neurologic/mental status: date and results of screenings for development/vision/hearing/speech; learning difficulty, seizure activity, clumsiness/falling, inappropriate behavior, tics, nervousness, night terrors/sleep walking
2. Geriatric
    a. General: unexplained weight change, change in ADL ability, change in heat/cold tolerance, increase in weakness, fatigue
    b. Head and neck: dizzy spells, headache, hair/skin changes, stiffness/limited ROM of neck, thyroid enlargement

    c. Eyes: change in visual acuity/field of vision/night vision, halo effect, increase in floaters, increased/decreased tearing, hx of cataract/glaucoma, date and result of last vision exam/last glaucoma test

    d. Ears: change in hearing acuity, use of and satisfaction with aid, change in cerumen characteristics, itching, vertigo, date and result of last hearing test

    e. Nose/sinuses: change in sense of smell, nasal obstruction, increase/decrease in nasal discharge, frequency of sinus pain/postnasal drip

    f. Mouth/throat: change in taste sensation, drying/cracking of lips and corners of mouth, dentition, use of and satisfaction with dentures, gum tenderness/bleeding/recession, bad breath/taste in mouth, sore tongue, increase/decrease in salivation, lesions, voice change, sore throat, difficulty chewing/swallowing

    g. CV: attention to all questions from Review of Systems (ROS): note recent changes and current medications in particular

    h. Respiratory: change in breathing characteristics (rate, depth, ease, comfort), SOB, cough, sputum

    i. Breast: changes in size, lumps, practice of self-breast exam, most recent mammography, breast enlargement in males

    j. GI: change in food tolerance/appetite, increased belching, change in bowel habits, hemorrhoids, increase in flatulence, use of laxative, date of last stool occult blood test, date of last proctoscopic exam

    k. GU: flank pain, change in urine characteristics or urination pattern, incontinence/dribbling, frequency/nocturia, satisfaction with level of sexual activity
       Females: menopause hx, vaginal lubrication, painful intercourse, treatment/medication post-menopause, last exam/Pap
       Males: prostatic pain/mass, change in erection/ejaculation

    l. Musculoskeletal (MSK): pain/stiffness/limited movement of joints/muscles, night cramping/twitching in legs, decreased hand strength/movement

    m. Endocrine: all questions from ROS are especially significant to elderly

    n. Hematopoietic/lymphatic: changes in diet, increased fatigue/pallor, increased bleeding/bruising tendency, enlarged/tender lymph nodes

    o. Integument: changes in moisture/texture/color/pigmentation/temperature, changes in moles/masses/rashes, pruritis, increased/decreased sensation, change in hair amount/texture/distribution, thickening/brittleness/softening of nails

    p. Immunologic: any recent changes in ROS data

    q. Neurologic/mental status: change in speech/memory/written or verbal communication, confusion, disorientation, decreased coordination/balance, tremors/tics/paralysis

3. Ethnic: be aware of race/culture-specific risk factors and ascertain individual client's status during ROS

Points to Remember

Integrate and organize questions from a variety of physiologic systems so that a cephalocaudal approach is used. This makes sense to clients and facilitates active client participation.

Assure client of the importance of the Review of Systems to enhance participation.

Each bit of data is important in the Review of Systems: use a checklist to ensure none are omitted.

Refer back to Review of Systems findings during the physical assessment and elicit further client information to ensure correlation of subjective and objective data.

Glossary

ADL (activities of daily living)—activities necessary to maintain an independent daily life, such as self-care, housekeeping, mobility, hygiene, etc.

Cephalocaudal—relating to the long axis of the body. Although literally translated as head-to-tail, the more common meaning is head-to-toe.

Crepitation—noise on movement

Hematopoietic—referring to blood and the formation of blood

Integument—the covering layer of the body, including skin, mucous membranes, hair, nails

Examiner's General Objective Assessment of Health Status

Learning Objectives

After studying this section, the reader should be able to:

- Describe the purposes of an initial general assessment.

- Gather information about client health status from observation, measurement, and screening.

- Record data in meaningful, objective terms.

V. Examiner's General Objective Assessment of Health Status

A. Definition: Global objective assessment data the caregiver gathers about the client's health before the actual physical examination

B. Purposes
1. Provides collectible, significant, objective data about health status before systematic physical exam
2. May provide clues to specific concerns noted in health history
3. Provides a comfortable transition from history-taking to physical exam

C. Initial impressions: data that can be gathered from observing the client during the introductory and history-taking period
  1. General appearance
     a. Presence or absence of all structures or obvious deformity
     b. Presence or absence of apparent distress/pain
     c. Appropriateness of dress
     d. Well-nourished/obese/emaciated
     e. Weight proportionate to height
     f. Size proportionate to age
     g. Normalcy of respiratory rate, rhythm, and ease
     h. Presence or absence of body odor
  2. Behavioral observations
     a. Appropriateness of behavior (if a child, include developmental appropriateness)
     b. If accompanied by a parent or significant other, appropriateness of client/significant other relationship
     c. Orientation to time, place, person
     d. Intactness of recent and remote memory
     e. Appropriateness of eye contact with caregiver (if a child, include appropriateness with parent)
  3. Affect—descriptors arranged on a continuum
     a. Happy .... sad
     b. Talkative ....quiet
     c. Animated ....depressed
     d. Mellow ....angry
     e. Relaxed .... tense/anxious
     f. Alert/focused ....distracted
  4. Sensory
     a. Obvious visual problem and/or wearing corrective lenses
     b. Obvious hearing problem and/or wearing hearing aid
     c. Obvious speech defect
     d. Ability to communicate in English
  5. Musculoskeletal
     a. Ability to move without stiffness, weakness, hesitation
     b. Ability to change position easily

      c. Ability to ambulate independently without unsteadiness or use of an assisting device

      d. Involuntary tremors or jerking of extremities and head

6. Skin

      a. Cyanosis or ruddiness of skin, mucous membranes, and/or sclera

      b. Facial paleness or flush, where able to distinguish

      c. Diaphoresis

      d. Visible lesions, rash, scars, significant nevi, varicosities

      e. Apparent edema of extremities or face

      f. Apparent ridged/ragged nails, clubbing, cyanotic nail beds

D. Measurements/vital signs: can be done initially or during system exam. Familiar, non-threatening procedures help acquaint client with caregiver's style and touch

1. Height
2. Weight
3. For children age 2 and under, head circumference
4. Temperature

      a. May be taken only if illness is suspected, or universally to determine baseline measurement

      b. For children too young for oral temperature measurement, some caregivers use axillary measurement; others prefer rectal. Take rectal temperature later in exam to avoid upsetting the child

5. Radial pulse: note rate, regularity, and quality
6. Respirations: note rate, regularity, ease, depth
7. Initial blood pressure: child seated

E. Screenings (See Section I for a list of screenings)

1) person
2) place
3) time
4) event

} abt oriented x

Points to Remember

The initial impressions are objective observations made while completing other aspects of the health assessment.

The system-by-system physical assessment will be more focused if preceded by a detailed subjective and general objective data bases.

Collecting general data and conducting familiar procedures at the beginning of the exam relaxes the client.

Initial impressions should be recorded as precise descriptors.

Glossary

Affect—outward expression of feeling or emotion

Descriptor—a word or phrase communicating a verbal picture

Head and Neck Assessment

Learning Objectives

After studying this section, the reader should be able to:

- Describe the structures and functions of major components of the head and neck.

- Examine the head and neck, using techniques of inspection, palpation, and auscultation.

- Identify age and ethnic variations in findings.

VI. Head and Neck Assessment

A. External structures of face

1. Shape and facial features vary with race
2. Facial expressions reveal affect of client
3. Trigeminal nerve (cranial nerve [CN] V) mediates sensation on face
4. Facial nerve (CN VII) regulates muscles used for facial expression

B. Internal structures of head and neck

1. Skull (see figures below)
   a. Protects brain
   b. Formed by several long plates joined by suture lines

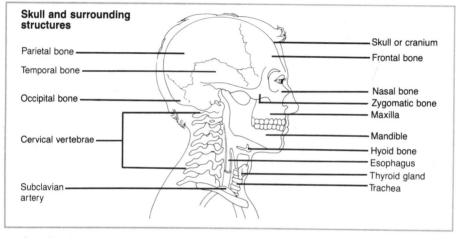

Skull and surrounding structures

Parietal bone
Temporal bone
Occipital bone
Cervical vertebrae
Subclavian artery

Skull or cranium
Frontal bone
Nasal bone
Zygomatic bone
Maxilla
Mandible
Hyoid bone
Esophagus
Thyroid gland
Trachea

2. Cervical spine: stabilizes head and neck
3. Musculature of neck: provides mobility for head and neck (see figure below)

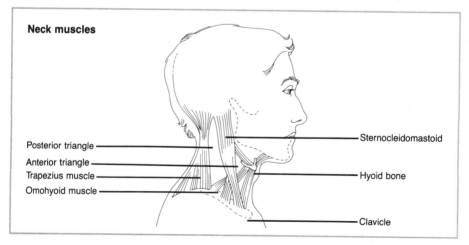

Neck muscles

Posterior triangle
Anterior triangle
Trapezius muscle
Omohyoid muscle

Sternocleidomastoid
Hyoid bone
Clavicle

4. Midline structures
   a. Trachea: major airway into bronchial tree
   b. Thyroid gland: only endocrine gland that can be examined directly
5. Lymph nodes of head and neck (see figure below)
   a. Drain head, ear, nose, sinuses and throat
   b. Produce lymphocytes
   c. Produce antibodies
   d. Perform phagocytosis

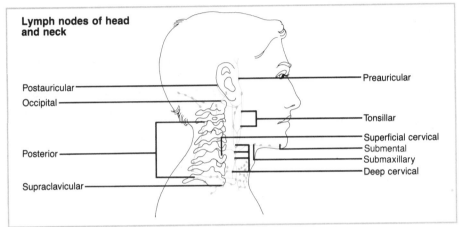

Lymph nodes of head and neck

Postauricular
Occipital
Posterior
Supraclavicular

Preauricular
Tonsillar
Superficial cervical
Submental
Submaxillary
Deep cervical

6. Great vessels of neck: blood supply for neck and head
   a. Internal and external jugular veins
   b. Carotid arteries

C. Inspection of head, face, and neck: normal findings
1. Skull should be symmetrical and without lesions
2. Facial structures should be symmetrical, not cyanotic, and without vascular lesions
3. Affect of patient should be observable through facial expression
4. Facial structures should be in proportion to one another
5. Trachea should be at midline position
6. Thyroid should not be observable
7. Range of motion of neck should be without limitation

D. Palpation of head, face, and neck: normal findings
1. Head should be free of lumps, tenderness
2. Strength of face muscles should be symmetrical, indicating adequate function of CN V and VII
3. Facial sensation should be symmetrical when stroking wisp of cotton on each cheek
4. Cervical spine should be free from crepitus, tenderness, lesions
5. Muscle strength in neck should be symmetrical

6. Client should shrug shoulders to test function of CN XI
7. Trachea should be midline and free from tenderness
8. Thyroid should be palpable but non-tender, symmetrical, free from lesions
9. Carotid arteries should have symmetrical quality in palpable pulse
10. Check lymph nodes. Normal findings include nodes that are
    a. Less than 1 cm in size
    b. Non-tender
    c. Good mobility
    d. Soft and discrete

E. Age and ethnic considerations
1. Pediatric
    a. Sutures and fontanel should be inspected and palpated in infants age 18 months and under
    b. Head circumference should be measured in children age 2 and under
    c. Lymph nodes are normally palpable in children because of lymphadenosis
2. Geriatric
    a. Great vessels may have bruits
    b. Quality of pulses in great vessels less
3. Ethnic variations
    a. Facial features such as epicanthal folds vary in form
    b. Head circumference is 1 to 2 cm smaller in Asians and Blacks

Points to Remember

Skull should be inspected and palpated for symmetry, lesions.

Facial structures should be observed for symmetry and alignment; for example, the eyes should align with tragus of ears.

Thyroid, the largest endocrine gland in the body, should be palpated and inspected for size, lesions, tenderness.

Glossary

Bruit—murmur heard over peripheral vessels

Lymphadenosis—hypertrophy or proliferation of lymph tissue

Eye Assessment

Learning Objectives

After studying this section, the reader should be able to:

- Identify the eye's major extraocular and intraocular structures and functions.

- List the steps of an eye exam.

- Describe normal anatomic and physiologic findings made during the examination.

- Use inspection and palpation to perform each step of the eye examination.

- Describe age and ethnic differences in technique and findings for the eye exam.

VII. Eye Assessment

A. External anatomic structures and physiologic functions

1. Orbit: cavity formed by frontal maxillary, zygomatic, lacrimal, sphenoid, ethmoid, and palatine bones
    a. The eye occupies anterior position of the orbit
    b. Posterior portion is composed of nerves, adipose tissue, and blood vessels to cushion eye
2. Muscles: six for each eye (see figure below)
    a. Four rectus muscles: superior, inferior, medial, and lateral; move eye in direction which names indicate
    b. Two oblique muscles: superior and inferior; rotate eyeball on axis
    c. All six muscles hold eyes parallel and create binocular vision
    d. Muscle function is governed by innervation of cranial nerves (CN) III (oculomotor), IV (trochlear), and VI (abducens)

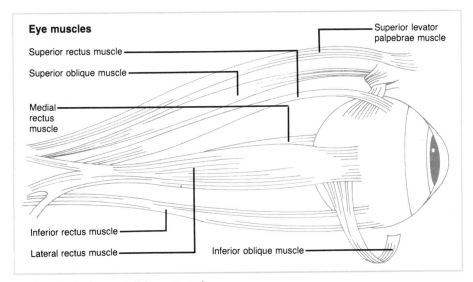

Eye muscles

Superior rectus muscle

Superior oblique muscle

Medial rectus muscle

Superior levator palpebrae muscle

Inferior rectus muscle

Lateral rectus muscle

Inferior oblique muscle

3. Eyelashes and lids protect the eye
    a. Palpebral fissure: space between the lids
    b. Lateral and medial canthi: point where upper and lower lids meet
    c. Tarsal plate: thin strips of connective tissue that lie within the lid and give it form
    d. Epicanthal folds: vertical folds of skin covering inner canthi
4. Lacrimal apparatus: keeps conjunctiva and cornea moist by secreting tears (see figure, next page)
    a. Lacrimal gland: located above and slightly lateral to eye; secretes tears
    b. Punctae: located on nasal end of upper and lower lid; drains tears
    c. Lacrimal sac and duct: collect tears and drain them into nose
5. Conjunctiva: thin transparent membrane lining each eyelid and anterior surface of eyes

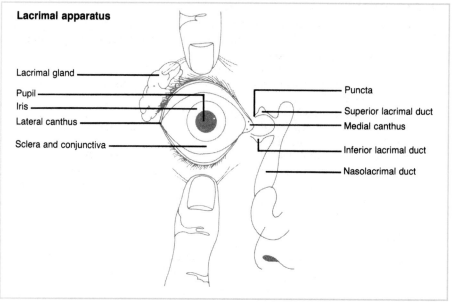

Lacrimal apparatus

Lacrimal gland

Pupil

Iris

Lateral canthus

Sclera and conjunctiva

Puncta

Superior lacrimal duct

Medial canthus

Inferior lacrimal duct

Nasolacrimal duct

    a. Bulbar conjunctiva: covers the sclera; contains many small blood vessels
    b. Palpebrae conjunctiva: recesses into folds of eyelids
    c. Caruncle: fleshy elevation set at nasal corner of conjunctiva
 6. Sclera: protects and supports eye
 7. Cornea: moist, transparent tissue covering pupil and iris; entry point for light
    a. Sensation caused by ophthalmic branch of CN V (Trigeminal)
    b. Blink reflex caused by stimulation of cornea and CN VIII (Facial)
 8. Anterior chamber: area between cornea and iris that contains fluid and aqueous humor, and regulates intraocular pressure
    a. Resistance to outflow of aqueous humor at anterior chamber angle increases intraocular pressure
    b. Ciliary body: produces aqueous humor
 9. Iris: colored portion; contains a circular muscle to regulate amount of light entering eye; analogous to diaphragm of camera
10. Pupil: the hole in the center of the iris that allows entrance of light; analogous to aperture of camera
    a. Size of pupil regulated by autonomic nervous system
    b. Amount of light influences size; pupils dilate in dim light, constrict in bright
11. Lens: found directly behind pupil
    a. Transparent and focuses light on the retina
    b. Ciliary body controls thickness of the lens, enabling eye to focus on far and near objects

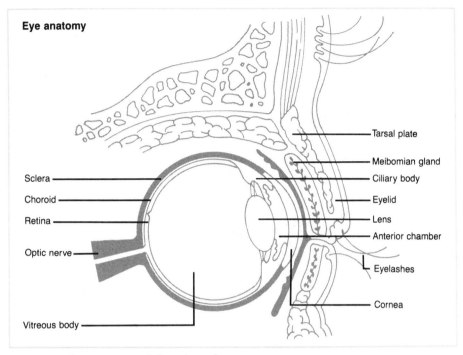

Eye anatomy

- Tarsal plate
- Meibomian gland
- Ciliary body
- Eyelid
- Lens
- Anterior chamber
- Eyelashes
- Cornea

- Sclera
- Choroid
- Retina
- Optic nerve
- Vitreous body

B. Internal anatomy and function of eye

1. Vitreous body: transparent fluid filled portion lying between the lens and the choroid
2. Choroid: thin vascular membrane on which the retina lies
3. Retina: observable only with ophthalmoscope; contains optic nerve and blood vessels
   a. Uniformly reddish orange in color
   b. Optic disc: head of optic nerve responsible for transmitting visual image to brain (CN II)
   c. Physiologic cup: small depression temporal to center of disk; indicator of intracranial pressure
   d. Retinal vessels: four sets of arteries and veins that nourish the retina; indicative of vascular health
   e. Fovea centralis: slight depression in retina; central point of vision; greatest color perception
   f. Macula: slightly darker colored retinal area immediately around fovea

C. Overview of eye assessment

1. Inspection and palpation of ocular structures
2. Testing of visual acuity and visual fields; inspection
3. Testing of ocular mobility; inspection
4. Ophthalmoscopic exam of internal structures; inspection

D. **Inspection and palpation of external structures** (examiner stands directly in front of client)

1. Inspection of eyelids, lashes, eyebrows and globe (eyeball): Normal findings
   a. Eyelids completely cover cornea when closed; no edema present
   b. Color corresponds to skin color
   c. Palpebral fissures are of equal height
   d. Margin of upper lid should fall between superior pupil margin and superior limbus; should be free from lesions such as a hordeolum or chalazion; should be symmetrical and without lag or droop when opened
   e. Eyelashes should be evenly distributed and curve outward
   f. Globe of eye should not protrude or be sunken into orbit
   g. Eyebrows should be of equal quantity, color and distribution
2. Palpation of eyelids and globe: procedure and normal findings
   a. Examiner places tips of index fingers on lids over sclera while client looks down
   b. Eyelids should not be tender or edematous
   c. Globes should feel equally firm without sponginess or hardness
3. Inspection of conjunctiva and sclera: procedure and normal findings
   a. Examiner separates lids widely while client looks down and then to each side
   b. Conjunctiva should be clear with small blood vessels visible
   c. Conjunctiva should be free from drainage
   d. White sclera should be visible through conjunctiva
4. Inspection of cornea and anterior chamber: normal findings
   a. Cornea should appear transparent, smooth and bright
   b. No irregularities or lesions should be visible
   c. Corneal sensitivity test of CN V: lids of both eyes should close when each cornea is stroked with wisp of cotton
   d. Anterior chamber transparent, free from visible material while inspected with oblique light from penlight
5. Inspection and palpation of lacrimal apparatus: normal findings
   a. No exudate, swelling or excessive tearing should be visible
   b. Palpation reveals lacrimal sac by pressing finger against lower inner orbital rim: no fluid regurgitation should occur through punctae
6. Inspection of iris: normal findings—symmetrical shape and color in both eyes
7. Inspection of pupils and pupillary responses: Procedure and normal findings
   a. Examiner observes accommodation response by having client shift gaze from a distant to a near object: eyes converge, pupils constrict, lenses thicken
   b. Examiner observation of pupillary response tests function of CN II and CN III
   c. Examiner uses a penlight to test pupillary response to light
   d. Pupils should be equal in size and shape
   e. Pupils should constrict equally when penlight beam is shined directly onto them (direct response)

    f. Opposite pupil should constrict when penlight is shined on one pupil (consensual response)

E. Testing visual acuity and visual fields
1. Visual acuity: procedure and normal findings
   a. Examiner tests each eye separately and both eyes together, with and without corrective lenses if client has them
   b. Examiner screens near vision with hand held card of newsprint; inability to read newsprint may indicate hyperopia in client under age 40 or presbyopia in client over age 40
   c. Acuity should be 20/20 in clients over age 8 using Snellen Chart at 20 feet (6 m)
   d. The larger the denominator, the poorer the vision; results other than 20/20 may indicate myopia
2. Visual fields: procedure and normal findings
   a. Examiner and client cover opposite eyes with opaque card
   b. Client should be able to visualize an object above, below, and from each side at the same time as examiner visualizes the object

F. Assessing ocular motility
1. Corneal light reflex
   a. Assesses alignment of anterior/posterior axes of the two eyes
   b. Bright dot of light from penlight held 12″ to 15″ (30 to 38 cm) from client should be at same spot on each cornea
2. Six cardinal positions of gaze
   a. Assess function of six ocular muscles and CN III, IV, and VI
   b. Eyes should move in parallel fashion in each of the six positions
   c. Eyes should be free of nystagmus
3. Cover/uncover test
   a. Assesses fusion and binocularity
   b. Uncovered eye should remain stable when looking at a penlight while other eye is covered
   c. Covered eye should be steady when cover is removed

G. Ophthalmoscopic inspection of internal structures
1. Principles of ophthalmoscopic exam
   a. Room light should be dimmed or off
   b. Lens selector is moved to accommodate for refractive error of examiner
   c. Examiner holds ophthalmoscope in his right hand to examine client's right eye
   d. Examiner holds his head about 1½ ft (0.5 m) in front of and about 15 degrees temporal to client's right line of vision
   e. Examiner's right index finger rests on lens selector dial to change it as necessary
   f. Examiner instructs client to look at a fixed point

g. Examiner finds optic disc by locating an optic vessel and following it in a nasal direction
2. Inspection of red reflex: normal findings—no clouding and opacity are present
3. Inspection of optic disc: normal findings
   a. Disc has orange-red appearance
   b. Disc margins are distinct
   c. Physiologic cup is visible and yellow-white
4. Inspecting retinal vessels: normal findings
   a. Arterioles are light red
   b. Arterioles are two-thirds the diameter of veins
   c. Arterioles have bright light reflex
   d. Veins are dark red
   e. Veins larger than arteries
   f. Veins have no light reflex
   g. Arteriole-venous crossing should be visible and without narrowing or lesions

H. Age and ethnic variation and strategies
1. Pediatric
   a. Visual acuity exam not possible in children under age 3
   b. Ophthalmoscopic exam not done in children under age 6 because they can't fixate on one point long enough
   c. Children age 7 and under normally have 20/30 visual acuity
   d. Tumble E or screening test such as Denver Eye Screening or Allen Picture Cards are used to examine acuity of preschoolers and toddlers
   e. A brightly-colored toy or puppet facilitates assessment of ocular mobility in infants and preschoolers
2. Geriatric
   a. Faulty position of eyelids, such as entropion, is common in the elderly from progressive relaxation of lid muscles
   b. A thin, grayish-white ring at the margin of the cornea, called arcus senilis, is normal in the elderly
   c. Eye may appear dry since lacrimal glands produce fewer tears
   d. Cornea clouds with aging
   e. Loss of peripheral vision is common
   f. Ophthalmoscopic exam shows mildly narrowed vessels and granular pigment in macula
3. Ethnic
   a. Small dark-pigmented dots may be visible on sclera near limbus in Blacks or dark-complected persons
   b. Oriental persons have epicanthic folds or folds of skin covering inner canthus

Points to Remember

Anatomy and physiology of eye is complex and requires several types of assessment.

External structures of the eyes should be clear and bright, symmetric, free from drainage, with pupils of equal size, reactivity to light, and accommodation ability.

An ophthalmoscope is used to examine the inner structures of the eye and to visualize the retina, the retinal vessels, and the red reflex.

Age and ethnic variations should be taken into account during eye exams.

Glossary

Aqueous humor—fluid secreted in ciliary body and found in the anterior and posterior chambers of the eye

Arcus senilis—gray to white opaque ring surrounding the cornea in individuals over age 50

Chalazion—sebaceous cyst on the eyelid formed by distention of meibomian gland with secretion

Hordeolum—inflammation of a sebaceous gland of the eyelid; sty

Hyperopia—faulty near vision

Myopia—faulty distance vision

Nystagmus—involuntary, rhythmic motion of the eye; may be horizontal, vertical, rotary, or mixed

Presbyopia—defect of vision in advancing age due to loss of elasticity of crystalline lens

Ear Assessment

Learning Objectives

After studying this section, the reader should be able to:

• Identify and explain the purposes of the major structures of the ear.

• Identify the major landmarks of the external ear and the tympanic membrane.

• Examine the external ear, mastoid process, and related lymphatic tissue, using inspection and palpation.

• Perform an otoscopic examination of the ear canal and tympanic membrane.

• Perform a gross hearing evaluation.

VIII. Ear Assessment

A. The major structures of the ear are diagrammed below

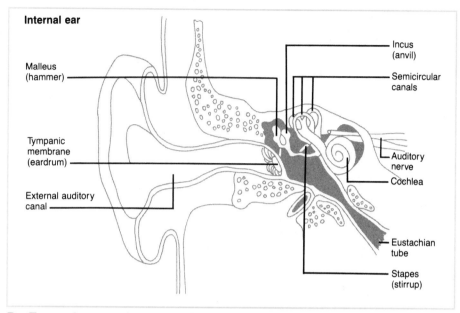

Internal ear

Malleus (hammer)

Tympanic membrane (eardrum)

External auditory canal

Incus (anvil)

Semicircular canals

Auditory nerve

Cochlea

Eustachian tube

Stapes (stirrup)

B. External ear structures and functions
  1. Auricle or pinna
     a. A multi-curved cartilaginous structure
     b. A sound wave collector
     c. Visible anatomic landmarks of the auricle

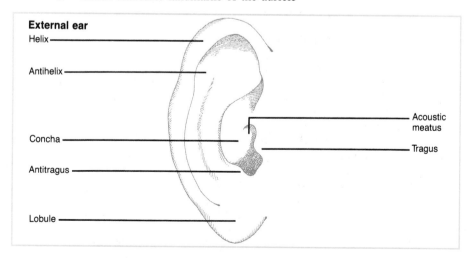

External ear

Helix

Antihelix

Concha

Antitragus

Lobule

Acoustic meatus

Tragus

2. External auditory canal
   a. S-shaped 1-in (2.5-cm) meatus extending from auricle to middle ear
   b. A sound wave transmitter
   c. External third is formed by cartilage; internal two thirds, by bone

C. Middle ear structures and functions
1. Tympanic membrane
   a. Translucent, gray membrane separating middle from external ear
   b. Vibratory membrane acts as a sound wave transmitter
   c. Visible anatomic landmarks of the tympanic membrane (TM)

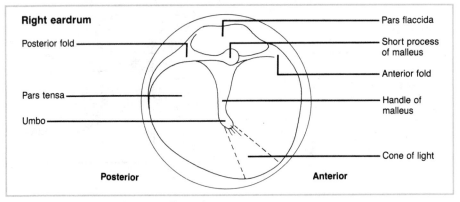

2. The bony ossicles: malleus, incus, stapes
   a. All three carry the tympanic membrane vibrations to the inner ear
   b. Malleus is connected to the tympanic membrane
   c. Stapes is connected to the oval window
3. Eustachian tube: equalizes air pressure in the middle ear and prevents rupture of the tympanic membrane

D. Inner ear structures and functions
1. Cochlea: the essential organ of hearing
   a. A fluid-filled coiled structure
   b. Sound waves stimulate sensory endings of the cochlear branch of CN VIII, resulting in hearing
2. Semicircular canals: the essential organ of balance
   a. Three fluid-filled curved structures
   b. Agitation in the fluid caused by movement stimulates sensory endings of the vestibular branch of CN VIII to maintain balance

E. Structures and functions of related areas
1. Regional lymph nodes
   a. Pre-auricular nodes are found anterior to the ear and postauricular nodes behind the ear
   b. Nodes drain part of the face, scalp, eyes, and external ear

2. Mastoid process
   a. Conical projection of the posterior portion of each temporal bone; extends downward behind the auricle
   b. Although part of skull, the mastoid process is important to ear exam; it can become inflamed by otitis media

F. Inspection
1. Auricle: procedure and normal findings
   a. Examiner faces client: the ears will be bilaterally symmetrical, proportionately sized, and have a vertical measurement between 1½" and 4" (4 cm and 10 cm)
   b. Examiner faces client's side: tip of ear will cross eye-occiput line (an imaginary line extending from the lateral aspect of the eye to the occipital protuberance), and long axis of the ear will be vertical or no more than 10 degrees from vertical to the eye-occiput line
   c. Color should match facial skin
   d. No sign of inflammation, lesions, or nodules should be present
   e. No visible discharge from canal should be present
   f. When auricle is bent forward, there should be no cracking, thickening, scaling, or lesions behind ear
   g. The external meatus should be patent
2. Auricular lymph nodes: normal findings
   a. Skin color should match surrounding area
   b. No redness or swelling should appear over nodes
3. Mastoid process: normal findings
   a. Skin color should match surrounding areas
   b. No redness or swelling should appear

G. Palpation
1. Auricle: normal findings
   a. No masses or tenderness during palpation
   b. No tenderness during manipulation of auricle and tragus
2. Auricular lymph nodes: normal findings
   a. Nodes small or not palpable
   b. If palpable, nodes discrete, mobile, non-tender
3. Mastoid process: normal findings
   a. No tenderness
   b. Bony edges of process well-defined

H. Principles of the otoscopic exam
1. Purpose of the otoscope: to see the auditory canal and TM
2. Otoscope light source should give off white, not yellow, light
3. Largest speculum that will fit into auditory canal comfortably yet be snug enough to provide seal for mobility testing is used
4. Handle of otoscope can be held in upright or downward position but must allow examiner's hand to be braced against client's head

5. Examiner holds otoscope in the dominant hand regardless of ear being examined
6. Procedure
   a. Examiner is facing and slightly above the client's side
   b. Client tilts head toward shoulder away from examiner
   c. Examiner pulls auricle upward and back to straighten canal
   d. Bony two-thirds of canal is very tender; use speculum with care
   e. Examiner watches as the speculum is inserted to avoid touching inflamed areas, lesions, etc.

I. Otoscopic inspection
   1. External auditory canal: normal findings
      a. Cerumen (ear wax): varied amount, consistency, and color
      b. Canal skin intact and uniformly pink
      c. No atresia of the canal
      d. No lesions, inflammation, tenderness, growths, discharge, or foreign bodies
   2. Tympanic membrane (TM): normal findings
      a. TM intact, without scars
      b. TM pearly gray, translucent, and shiny, with a light reflex present from about 5:00 to 7:00
      c. Landmarks visible, but not exaggerated
      d. No fluid, bubbles, pus, or blood seen through TM
      e. TM moves when air is blown into canal through the insufflating device, or when client blows gently with nostrils pinched and lips closed

J. Hearing evaluation: provides gross assessment of hearing acuity, testing cochlear branch of auditory cranial nerve VIII
   1. Whisper test
      a. Test evaluates higher range acuity
      b. Client will hear softly whispered words at 1 ft to 2 ft (0.3 to 0.6 m) with opposite ear occluded
      c. Results will be bilaterally equal
   2. Watch tick test (optional)
      a. Test evaluates higher frequency acuity
      b. Client will hear ticking watch 1" to 2" (2.5 to 5 cm) from auditory meatus with opposite ear occluded
      c. Results will be bilaterally equal
   3. Rinne test
      a. Test compares air to bone conduction, to detect conduction deficit
      b. A tuning fork of more than 500 cps is used
      c. Examiner strikes fork, places end of handle on mastoid process; when client no longer hears tone, examiner moves fork so prongs are in front of meatus; asks client if he/she hears sound and, if so, when it stops (some examiners then assess how much longer they hear tone)

    d. Air conduction in hearing acute subject remains audible twice as long as bone conduction (record as AC > BC)

4. Weber test
   a. Test detects conduction deficit and/or sensory neural deficit
   b. A tuning fork of more than 500 cps is used
   c. Examiner smartly strikes fork, places base on midline of forehead or top of skull; asks client where he/she hears the sound
   d. A hearing acute client hears sound all over in the head or equally in both ears (no lateralization)
   e. Client hearing sound in right ear has either right-sided conduction deficit or left-sided sensorineural deficit
   f. If client has a known unilateral loss, sound is heard in affected ear if there is conductive deficit and unaffected (or less affected) ear if a sensorineural deficit

K. Age and ethnic variations and strategies

1. Pediatric
   a. Small children should be held by adult during otoscopic assessment to allow the examiner good visualization and prevent client discomfort or injury from head movement
   b. If possible, examine ears while child is quiet; crying increases pressure on and blood flow to the TM, often turning it temporarily pink
   c. Ear canal in child age 3 and under has upward curvature; auricle must be pulled downward and out for visualization
   d. Assessment of pinna position is essential in infants because of relationship to developmental disability
2. Geriatric
   a. Auricle loses elasticity, lobe may elongate and develop linear oblique wrinkles
   b. TM may lose mobility, increase in opacity, lose lustre
   c. Cerumen may be drier and harder
   d. Hair growth in auditory canal may be increased
   e. Senile atrophy of TM may make landmarks appear exaggerated
3. Ethnic
   a. Cerumen tends to be soft and moist, tan to brown in Caucasians and Blacks
   b. Cerumen tends to be dry and grayish in Native Americans and Orientals

Points to Remember

The auricle is manipulated differently for adults than for small children during otoscopic exams.

Normal cerumen can have a wide range of characteristics.

The hand that holds the otoscope must be braced against the client's head to prevent discomfort or injury.

TM color and the presence of a light reflex indicate the health of the auditory apparatus.

Hearing tests indicate the patency of cranial nerve VIII, the auditory nerve.

Glossary

Auricle or pinna—the cartilaginous structure forming the external, visible ear

Cerumen (ear wax)—a mixture of sebum and apocrine sweat from glands in the external auditory canal

Otoscope—the instrument used to visualize and illuminate the external auditory canal and tympanic membrane

Tympanic membrane—the thin, mobile layer of tissue that transmits sound waves from the external environment to the middle ear

Visible anatomic landmarks—points of reference: helpful in accurately describing assessment findings

Nose and Throat Assessment

Learning Objectives

After studying this section, the reader should be able to:

- Describe the structure and function of the nose and throat.

- Examine the nose and throat using inspection and palpation.

- List normal objective findings in anatomic and physiologic terms.

IX. Nose and Throat Assessment

A. External structure

1. Bridge: upper two thirds of nose supported by bone
2. Vestibule: opening that surrounds the nares
3. Columella: skin-covered cartilaginous structure that divides the vestibule
4. Septum: cartilaginous and bony structure that separates the nares; forms medial wall of nasal cavity

B. Internal structure

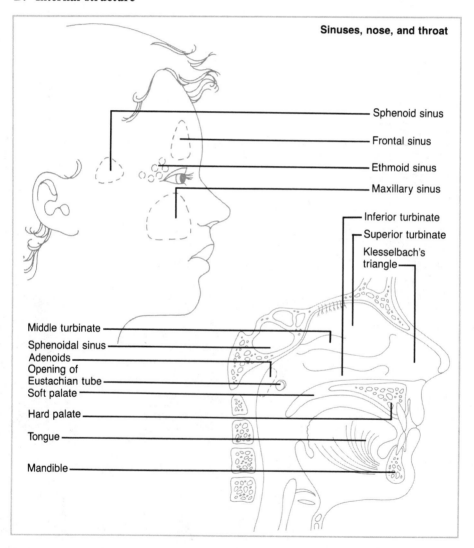

Sinuses, nose, and throat

Sphenoid sinus
Frontal sinus
Ethmoid sinus
Maxillary sinus
Inferior turbinate
Superior turbinate
Klesselbach's triangle
Middle turbinate
Sphenoidal sinus
Adenoids
Opening of Eustachian tube
Soft palate
Hard palate
Tongue
Mandible

1. Turbinates
   a. Superior
   b. Medial: can be seen by inspection
   c. Inferior: can be seen by inspection
2. Middle meatus: opening between superior and medial turbinate that drains the sinuses
3. Inferior meatus: drains the nose and lacrimal duct
4. Nasal mucosa: lining of nares covered with cilia; pinkish red due to rich vascular supply
5. Paranasal sinuses
   a. Sphenoid: in the middle of skull (visible only with X-ray)
   b. Ethmoid: behind the orbit of the eye (visible only with X-ray)
   c. Frontal: above eyebrow in each eye (visible only with X-ray)
   d. Maxillary: located along each maxilla; largest sinus; can hold up to 20 cc of fluid

C. **Functions of nose and sinuses**
   1. Mucosal cilia cleanses inspired air
   2. Nasal mucous membrane humidifies air
   3. Vascular supply warms inspired air
   4. Houses receptors for sense of smell; cranial nerve I

D. **Inspection of external structure of the nose: normal findings**
   1. Nose is symmetrical or without deviation of septum
   2. Nose free from lesions
   3. No flaring of nares
   4. Nose free from discharge
   5. Maxillary and frontal sinuses should be non-edematous
   6. Client should be able to identify familiar odors

E. **Palpation of external structures: normal findings**
   1. External nose free from structural deviation
   2. No tenderness
   3. No swelling
   4. Frontal and maxillary sinuses free from tenderness, swelling

F. **Inspection of internal structures: normal findings**
   1. Nasal mucosa pinkish red without purulent drainage
   2. No foreign bodies visible
   3. No lesions on nasal mucosa (e.g., polyps or ulcerations)
   4. No evidence of old blood

G. **Age and ethnic variations**
   1. Toddlers may have foreign bodies in nose
   2. Older adults have diminished sense of smell due to atrophy of olfactory nerve (CN I) fibers

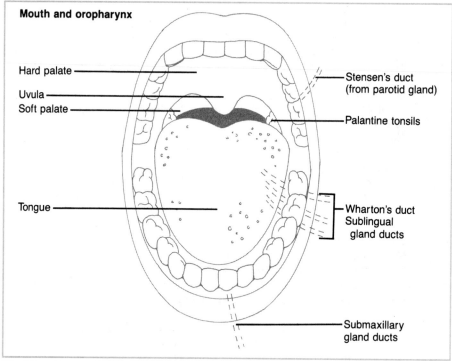

Mouth and oropharynx

Hard palate

Uvula

Soft palate

Tongue

Stensen's duct
(from parotid gland)

Palantine tonsils

Wharton's duct
Sublingual
gland ducts

Submaxillary
gland ducts

H. Structure and function of mouth and oropharynx
1. Cheek: contains buccinator muscle
2. Lips
3. Teeth: 32 in adult
4. Gingiva (gums): usually pink
5. Tongue
   a. Papillae: taste buds
   b. Innervated by CN XII for movement
   c. CN VII and IX: sensory receptors for taste
6. Buccal mucosa: pinkish red
7. Hard palate: white
8. Soft palate: pink; forms roof of oral cavity
9. Anterior and posterior pillars: form an arch in the mouth
10. Tonsils: located between anterior and posterior pillars; lymph tissue
11. Uvula: muscular tissue that hangs from posterior margins of soft palate
12. Mandible: forms bony framework of mouth
13. Temporomandibular joint: located 1 cm anterior to tragus of the ear
14. Openings to salivary glands
    a. Parotid (Stenson's) duct; opens into buccal membrane opposite second molar
    b. Submandibular (Wharton's) duct; side of frenulum on floor of mouth

    c. Sublingual: forms sublingual fold and has openings on this fold

15. Functions of the mouth
    a. First division of the digestive tube
    b. Entrance to respiratory system
    c. Conducts air to and from the larynx
    d. Cheeks contain muscles of mastication
    e. Mandible contributes to slope of face and mouth
    f. TM joint responsible for opening and closing mouth
    g. Teeth masticate food
    h. Salivary glands secrete saliva; enzyme in saliva begins digestive process
    i. Tongue assists in swallowing and in speech
    j. Hard and soft palate contribute to speech sounds

16. Oral receptors for cranial nerves V, VII, IX, X, XII
    a. V: controls masticator muscles
    b. VII: controls mastication and taste sensations
    c. IX: responsible for taste sensations and movement of pharynx
    d. X: causes gag reflex
    e. XII: responsible for tongue movement

17. Lips and facial structure: normal findings
    a. Lips free from dryness, cracking, or lesions
    b. Lips pink without cyanosis
    c. Facial structure symmetrical
    d. Client can easily open and close mouth
    e. Client can purse lips and puff out cheeks (CN VII motor branch)

18. Mucous membrane, teeth, gums, and tongue (anterior pharynx): normal findings
    a. Mucosa light pink and moist
    b. Mucosa free from ulcers or lesions
    c. Salivary ducts visible and free from inflammation
    d. Tongue pink, free from swelling, coating, ulcers, or lesions
    e. Tongue moves easily (CN XII) without tremor
    f. Teeth not missing or maloccluded
    g. Teeth free from caries or breakage
    h. Gums pink and free from tartar, inflammation, or hemorrhage

19. Hard and soft palate, arches, tonsils, uvula, posterior pharynx: normal findings
    a. Hard palate white
    b. Soft palate pink
    c. Anterior and posterior arches free from swelling and inflammation
    d. Posterior pharynx free from lesions and inflammation
    e. Uvula moves and gag reflex elicited with tongue blade on posterior pharynx (CN X)
    f. Tonsils right size for age, free from lesions

I. Palpation of oral structures: normal findings
1. TM joint free from tenderness and crepitus

2. Lips free from pain and induration
3. Posterior and lateral surfaces of tongue free from lesions, unusual color, tenderness, swelling
4. Floor of mouth free from tenderness, nodules, swelling
5. Teeth not loose or painful when palpated

J. Age and ethnic variations
  1. Pediatrics
     a. Lymph tissue proliferates through late school age so tonsils will be enlarged as compared to adult
     b. Primary teeth do not erupt until age 5 to 6 months, on average
     c. 20 primary teeth are present by age 2½
     d. Eruption of 32 permanent teeth not complete until late adolescence
     e. Tongue depressor is needed to examine mouth and throat of infants and small children; save this exam for last, since its discomfort can cause crying
     f. Yellow-white nodules may be found on palates of newborns and infants
  2. Geriatric
     a. Papillae atrophy on lateral tongue edges, reducing taste perception
     b. Salivary glands atrophy, drying the mucosal surfaces of mouth
     c. Older clients may have dentures (these must be removed before inspection of mouth)
  3. Ethnic variations
     a. Tongue and oral mucosa are usually dark in Blacks
     b. Bony growth on roof of mouth (tours palatinis) is often seen in Asians
     c. Native Americans may exhibit cleft uvula
     d. A grayish white lesion on buccal mucosa, called leukoedema, is often found in Blacks
     e. Native Americans and Asians often have congenital absence of third permanent molars

Points to Remember

Nose warms, humidifies, and cleans inspired air.

Sinuses and nasal lacrimal duct drain into openings between turbinates.

Mucous membrane of mouth should be pink, moist, and free from lesions.

Cranial nerves innervate the mouth, controlling tongue and nose and influencing taste, smell, tongue and masticator muscle movement, and the gag reflex.

Several age and ethnic variations influence the structure, function and examination techniques for the nose and mouth.

Glossary

Stensen's ducts—another name for the parotid duct; opens opposite the second molar

Wharton's duct—another name for submandibular duct; opens onto floor of mouth

Thorax and Lung Assessment

Learning Objectives

After studying this section, the reader should be able to:

- Identify the topographical landmarks of the thorax.

- Examine the respiratory system using inspection, palpation, percussion, and auscultation.

- Record objective data related to an examination.

- Recognize variations in technique and normal findings related to age and ethnicity.

X. Thorax and Lung Assessment

A. Topographical landmarks of thorax
1. Help examiner locate internal structures such as heart and lungs
2. Provide mechanisms for evaluating findings
3. Help describe findings

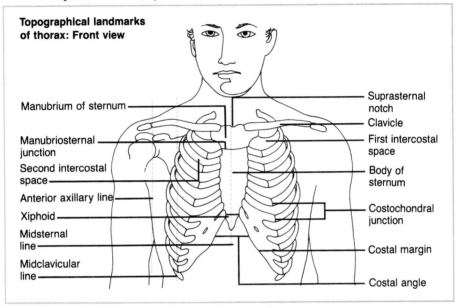

Topographical landmarks of thorax: Front view

- Manubrium of sternum
- Manubriosternal junction
- Second intercostal space
- Anterior axillary line
- Xiphoid
- Midsternal line
- Midclavicular line
- Suprasternal notch
- Clavicle
- First intercostal space
- Body of sternum
- Costochondral junction
- Costal margin
- Costal angle

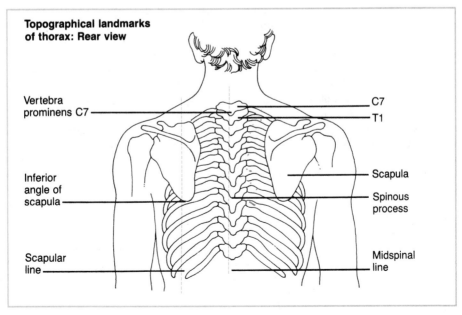

Topographical landmarks of thorax: Rear view

- Vertebra prominens C7
- Inferior angle of scapula
- Scapular line
- C7
- T1
- Scapula
- Spinous process
- Midspinal line

R - 3 lobe
L 2 lobes

B. Major anterior topographical landmarks
1. Manubriosternal junction (angle of Louis)
   a. Articulation point of second rib and upper sternum
   b. Useful in numbering ribs accurately
   c. Positioned a few centimeters below suprasternal notch
   d. Mid-sternal line: imaginary line from suprasternal notch to costal angle

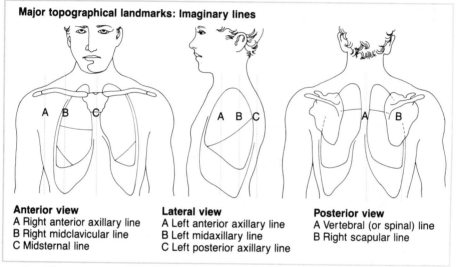

Major topographical landmarks: Imaginary lines

A B C   A B C   A   B

Anterior view
A Right anterior axillary line
B Right midclavicular line
C Midsternal line

Lateral view
A Left anterior axillary line
B Left midaxillary line
C Left posterior axillary line

Posterior view
A Vertebral (or spinal) line
B Right scapular line

2. Ribs
   a. First seven ribs articulate with the sternum at the costal cartilages
   b. Ribs 8, 9 and 10 articulate with above costal cartilages
   c. Intercostal spaces are numbered by the rib immediately above them
   d. Costal angle: formed by intersection of costal margins
3. Anterior and lateral landmarks
   a. Mid-clavicular lines (MCL): imaginary lines extending from midpoints of right and left clavicles parallel to mid-sternal line
   b. Anterior axillary lines: imaginary lines extending vertically from anterior axillary fold along anterior lateral chest wall right and left
   c. Mid-axillary lines: imaginary lines running right and left midway between anterior and posterior axillary lines

C. Major posterior thoracic landmarks
1. Right and left scapulae
2. Vertebra prominens: seventh cervical vertebrae
   a. Most prominent spinous process; best felt when client flexes neck
   b. Above T1
   c. Most helpful landmark in locating structure of posterior thorax; overlies first rib
3. Thoracic vertebrae; T5 adjacent to sixth rib
4. Mid-spinal line: vertical line along posterior spinous processes

5. Scapular lines: imaginary vertical lines passing through inferior angles of right and left scapulae
6. Posterior axillary lines: imaginary vertical lines running from right and left posterior axillary folds along posterolateral thorax wall

D. Underlying thoracic structures and their functions
1. Trachea: bifurcates at angle of Louis; large airway into bronchi
2. Main bronchi
   a. Large tube between tracheal bifurcation and lung tissue that allows air to enter lung
   b. Right mainstem bronchus larger than left
3. Bronchioles: intermediate-size airways between bronchi and alveoli
4. Lung borders
   a. Apices of lungs rise 2 to 4 cm above inner third of clavicle anteriorly
   b Each lung is divided in half by an oblique or major fissure which runs from T3 close to vertebral border of scapula posteriorly, and sixth rib at MCL anteriorly
   c. Right upper lobe divided from right middle lobe by horizontal fissure running from right mid-axillary line at the level of the fifth rib anteriorly across at the level of the fifth rib
5. Diaphragm
   a. Anteriorly, right dome of diaphragm is located at levels of fifth rib at MCL during expiration
   b. Anteriorly, left dome is at level of sixth rib during expiration
   c. Posteriorly, left dome is at T10 level and eighth rib during expiration

E. Inspection of thorax and respiratory effort
1. Preparation of client
   a. Ask client to sit upright without support
   b. Have client disrobe to waist
   c. Provide private room with good overhead lighting and adequate warmth
2. Configuration of chest: normal findings
   a. Symmetrical side to side
   b. Anteroposterior diameter is less than transverse diameter with a 1:2 to 5:7 ratio in an adult
   c. Not barrel shaped
   d. Free from kyphosis posteriorly _—humpback_
   e. Free from retraction
   f. Free from sternal protrusion (pectus carinatum)
   g. Sternum not depressed into thorax (pectus excavatum)
3. Ribs and interspaces: normal findings
   a. Free from retraction during inspiration
   b. Free from bulging during expiration
   c. Costal angle less than 90 degrees
   d. Ribs inserted into spine at 45 degree angle
   e. Barrel shape and greater angles may indicate obstructive lung disease

nail beds . filling 2 sec

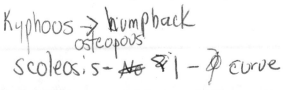

Kyphoos → humpback
osteopous
scoleosis - No 8°1 - Ø curve

4. Patterns of respiration: normal findings
   a. Men and children breathe diaphragmatically
   b. Women breathe thoracically
   c. Normal adult rate is 16-20/minute with regular rhythm
   d. Breathing should be free from distress (dyspnea)
5. Other areas affected by respiratory states: normal findings
   a. Lips free from cyanosis
   b. Fingers not clubbed — *longterm hypoxia*

F. Palpation of thorax
1. General palpation
   a. Skin warm and dry to touch anterior and posterior (A&P)
   b. Chest free of tenderness A&P
   c. Chest free of bulges A&P
   d. Muscle mass symmetrical A&P *excursion — expand equally*
2. Assessment of respiratory excursion: procedure and normal findings
   a. Examiner places thumbs anteriorly along costal margin and pushes toward xiphoid
   b. Examiner places palms posteriorly on lateral chest with thumbs at level of 10th rib
   c. Examiner's thumbs should move symmetrically on both sides as client inhales deeply
3. Assessment of fremitus (palpable vibrations transmitted through bronchopulmonary system to chest wall when client says one-two-three): procedure and normal findings
   a. Examiner uses palmar surfaces of fingers starting from apices, proceeding downard and comparing side to side anteriorly, laterally, and posteriorly
   b. Fremitus most intense at second intercostal space near bronchial bifurcation
   c. Fremitus decreased or absent with pleural effusion, pneumothorax, or obstruction of bronchus
   d. Fremitus increased in pneumonia or masses in lung

G. Percussion — *hit joint of middle finger 2 then move*
1. Technique
   a. Utilize mediate percussion (described in section I)
   b. Start at apices and proceed downward
   c. Compare side to side
   d. Percuss at 5 cm intervals
   e. Avoid bony prominences such as scapula
   f. Percuss in interspaces
   g. Note duration, pitch and tone
   h. Percussion note over normal lungs is resonance
2. Percuss level of diaphragmatic excursion
   a. Note change from resonance over normal lung to dullness over diaphragm

fremitus — palpate lung for vibration of thick secretions say "99"

b. Level of dullness slightly higher on right side
c. Measure and mark distance between level of dullness on full expiration and inspiration; normal finding is 5 to 6 cm

H. Auscultation
1. Technique
   a. Utilize diaphragm of stethoscope
   b. Have client breathe through mouth, a little more deeply than normal
   c. Watch for signs of hyperventilation such as light-headedness
   d. Place stethoscope firmly on skin; avoid moving over muscle and hair
   e. Listen to one complete respiratory cycle
   f. Utilize same sequence outlined under palpation and percussion
   g. Note quality and intensity of breath sounds
2. Normal auscultatory findings
   a. Vesicular sounds: heard over most lung tissue
   b. Bronchovesicular: heard over mainstem bronchi, between scapulae and below clavicles
   c. Bronchial: heard over trachea
3. Adventitious sounds
   a. Normal sound heard in wrong place, e.g., bronchovesicular sounds heard over most of lung instead of just bronchi
   b. Crackles (rales): discrete non-continuous crackling sound heard best with inspiration
   c. Rhonchi: high-pitched, continous wheezing sound heard with expiration; coughing may alter sound
   d. Friction rub: creaking or grating sound of inflamed surfaces rubbing together; coughing has no effect

I. Age and ethnic considerations
1. Pediatric
   a. Hyperresonance may be percussed over lungs of small infants
   b. Bronchovesicular breath sounds may be heard normally in small children
   c. Chest must be inspected carefully for deformities
2. Geriatric
   a. Kyphosis may be present from osteoporosis and collapse of vertebrae
   b. Chest wall less compliant
   c. Inspiration less deep
3. Ethnic: pigmentary demarcation lines along anterior chest in Orientals and Blacks

Dull / dense tissue – greater.
Flat / normal lung

Pensense → emphaysma

tympany → air

Points to Remember

Inspection, palpation, percussion, and auscultation are all utilized to perform a comprehensive respiratory assessment.

Percussion, palpation, and auscultation are conducted in the following order: top to bottom while comparing results side to side.

Imaginary lines and anatomical landmarks help locate and standardize findings.

The normal percussion note for the chest is resonance.

The majority of normal lung sounds are vesicular.

Bronchial sounds are auscultated over the trachea.

Bronchovesicular sounds are auscultated over the mainstem bronchi.

Glossary

Adventitious sounds—abnormal breath sounds heard with auscultation, including crackles, rhonchi, and friction rubs, as well as normal sounds heard in abnormal locations, e.g., bronchial over most of lung instead of trachea

Fremitus—a palpable vibration over thorax when client speaks

Friction rub—a crackling, grating sound heard through stethoscope when two inflamed surfaces rub together

Cardiovascular Assessment

Learning Objectives

After studying this section, the reader should be able to:

- Describe the basic structures and functions of the cardiovascular system.

- Explain the circulation of blood through the heart and body.

- Perform an assessment, using inspection, palpation, and auscultation of the heart and great vessels.

- Perform an assessment, using inspection, palpation, and auscultation of the peripheral vascular system.

- Record objective findings accurately and precisely.

XI. Cardiovascular Assessment

A. External structures and functions

1. Circulatory system is entirely internal but visible landmarks help locate internal structures
2. External anatomic landmarks (see figure below)

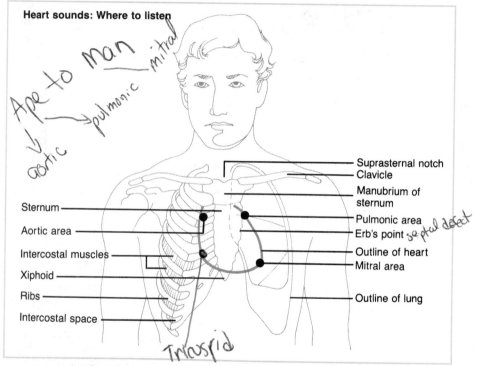

Heart sounds: Where to listen

[handwritten notes: Ape to man, → mitral, → pulmonic, aortic, Tricuspid, septal defect]

Labels (right side): Suprasternal notch, Clavicle, Manubrium of sternum, Pulmonic area, Erb's point, Outline of heart, Mitral area, Outline of lung

Labels (left side): Sternum, Aortic area, Intercostal muscles, Xiphoid, Ribs, Intercostal space

a. Aortic valve: best felt and heard at second right intercostal space adjacent to sternum
b. Pulmonary valve: best felt and heard at second left intercostal space adjacent to sternum
c. Tricuspid valve: best felt and heard at fifth left intercostal space adjacent to sternum
d. Mitral valve: best felt and heard at fifth left intercostal space just medial of the mid-clavicular line; over apex of heart and point of maximum impulse (PMI) *[handwritten: ~ 1 cm, about the size of finger pad]*
e. Mitral valve actually lies under left edge of sternum at third intercostal space (Erb's point)

B. Internal structures and functions

1. The heart and great vessels
   a. The heart is a pump designed to simultaneously receive and disgorge

both oxygenated and unoxygenated blood; its muscular structure, valves, and conductivity system enable it to do so

b. Cardiac circulation includes blood flow through heart and major vessels

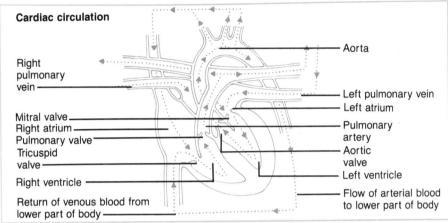

Cardiac circulation

Right pulmonary vein

Mitral valve
Right atrium
Pulmonary valve
Tricuspid valve

Right ventricle

Return of venous blood from lower part of body

Aorta

Left pulmonary vein
Left atrium

Pulmonary artery

Aortic valve
Left ventricle

Flow of arterial blood to lower part of body

c. Valves work uni-directionally to keep blood moving in the proper direction. Heart sounds are produced by valves closing; murmurs are heard when valves work inefficiently or close incompletely and allow back flow. Split sounds are heard when timing of valve closing is inexact

d. Right heart receives venous blood and pumps it through the pulmonary arteries to both lungs, where it is oxygenated

e. Left heart receives oxygenated blood from the lungs through the pulmonary veins; the blood is then pumped through the aorta to the entire body   *cor* p pulse

2. Cardiac cycle: systolic and diastolic phase

a. Systole: ventricles are full of blood and begin to contract. Tricupsid and mitral valves close, producing S1, first heart sound. Blood flows into arteries, decreasing ventricular pressure. Ventricles empty, pulmonary and aortic valves close (S2) beginning diastole   resting

b. Diastole: blood flows back into atria through veins and then through open mitral and tricuspid valves, refilling ventricles

c. Systole lasts one third of cycle and diastole two thirds

C. Structures and functions of the peripheral vascular system

1. Peripheral system is composed of vessels, arteries, capillaries, veins; carries oxygen and blood to body, then returns blood to lungs for reoxygenation

2. This system's health can be measured in several ways

a. When larger vessels come close to surface and overlie a bone, they can be assessed for patency, condition of vessel wall, and certain pulse characteristics

b. Systolic blood pressure measurement indicates amount of circulatory resistance within the arteries; diastolic blood pressure indicates stroke

volume and pressure exerted against arteries
   c. Externally visible and palpable characteristics of extremities reveal their level of oxygenation and ability of vascular system to circulate fluid

D. Inspection of precordium: Procedure and normal findings
1. Client lies supine or reclining at 45 degrees or less
2. Chest wall should not lift or heave with heart beat; pulsations should not be visible, except possibly at PMI

E. Palpation of precordium: Procedure and normal findings
1. Examiner palpates chest with palmar surfaces of fingers
2. Chest should not lift with heart beat
3. No thrills should be present
4. No pulsations, except PMI and epigastric area, should be present
   a. At PMI localized ($<\frac{1}{2}''$ or 1.25 cm diameter area) tapping pulse may be felt at start of systole
   b. In epigastric area (under edge of rib cage near base of sternum), pulsation from abdominal aorta may be palpable

F. Auscultation of precordium: procedure, normal findings, and abnormal findings
1. Examiner auscultates these areas, using bell and diaphragm: aortic, pulmonic, tricuspid, apical, and Erb's point
2. Examiner auscultates with client in three of the four following positions: sitting, supine, left lateral, sitting leaning forward
3. These sounds are normal:
   a. S1: a "lub" sound heard best over mitral area with bell in left lateral positions; longer, lower, and louder there than S2. Normal S1 splitting may be audible in tricuspid area
   b. S2: a "dub" sound heard best through diaphragm in aortic area with client sitting and leaning over; shorter, sharper, higher, and louder there than S1. Normal S2 splitting may be audible on inspiration in pulmonic area
   c. S3: may be normal in children and slender young adults with no cardiovascular pathology. S3 is sound of blood falling into empty ventricles after beginning of diastole. Heard best during expiration in mitral area with bell when client is supine; sounds short, dull, soft, low
   d. Murmurs may be functional in children and young adults. Innocent murmurs are soft, short, vary with respirations and position, occur in early systole, are heard best in pulmonic or mitral areas when client is supine
4. These sounds indicate need for diagnostic examination or referral:
   a. Fixed or widely-spaced S2 splitting
   b. S3 in older adults
   c. S4, a low-pitched sound in late diastole; heard best at apex
   d. Other sounds: "gallops" (loud S3 or S4 sounds); "clicks" or "snaps"

[handwritten margin notes: "Third heart sound"; "ventricular gallop / pathological"; "Atrial gallop"; "Atrial gallop"; "Allen test → cut of ulnar and radial artery et blanch out hand then release ulnar and hand should pink up."]

(produced by valves opening); friction rubs (rubbing of the pericardium)

   e. Murmurs: may occur in any valve; describe location and position where best heard, timing in the cardiac cycle, pitch, character, loudness (see below). Subjective grading scale for assessing murmurs:
   Grade I: soft, not heard every beat
   Grade II: soft, heard every beat
   Grade III: loud
   Grade IV: loud, with thrill – touch and wir brates.
   Grade V: very loud, with thrill
   Grade VI: audible with stethoscope off the chest

G. Inspection of peripheral vascular system: normal findings

1. Pulsation and/or distension of jugular vein may be seen in supine client
   a. Decreases with inspiration, increases with expiration
   b. Pulsation regular, diffuse
   c. Not present when client is sitting higher than at a 45 degree angle
2. Extremities
   a. Circulation intact, symmetrical and adequate for healthy integument; see Integument Section for criteria
   b. No pulsation visible
   c. No venous bulging or distension
   d. No edema

H. Palpation of peripheral vascular system: procedure and normal findings

1. Examiner palpates pulses in these arteries: carotid, temporal, brachial, radial, femoral, popliteal, dorsalis pedis, and posterior tibial
   a. Do not palpate both carotid arteries simultaneously; it may decrease blood supply to brain
   b. Femoral and radial pulses beat in synchrony
   c. Carotid and apical pulses beat in synchrony
   d. Dorsalis pedis and posterior tibial pulses may be absent
   e. Pulses will be present, regular, 60 to 90 beats/minute, not bounding or thready; symmetrical
   f. Arterial walls will feel soft, elastic
   g. Record by drawing stick figure; label sites using the following pulse rating:
   0 = absent; 1 + = barely perceptible (thready); 2 + = diminished; 3 + = normal; 4 + = bounding
2. Palpation of extremities will reveal symmetrically even temperature without edema, tenderness, or superficial veins

I. Auscultation of peripheral vascular system: procedure and normal findings

1. Examiner measures arterial blood pressure in both arms with client sitting
   a. Systolic should not exceed 140
   b. Diastolic should not exceed 90
   c. Pressure in arms should not vary more than 10 mg Hg

2. Examiner assesses pressure (both arms) with client standing if history of orthostatic hypotension or on anti-hypertensive medicine
   a. Systolic pressure should not drop >15 mm Hg
   b. Diastolic pressure should not drop >5 mm Hg
3. Examiner assesses pressure (both sides) in legs if femoral or popliteal pulses are weak or nonpalpable
   a. Systolic pressure should be higher than in arm
   b. Diastolic pressure should be the same or slightly lower
4. Examiner auscultates carotid and femoral arteries; should reveal no bruits

J. Age-related variations
   1. Pediatric
      a. Use small stethoscope to better localize sounds
      b. Sinus arrhythmia is common; time pulse with respirations. If child can hold breath, time while breath is held
      c. S2 may be heard best in pulmonic area
      d. S3 occurs normally in 30% of children
      e. Functional murmurs are common
      f. Pulse rate and blood pressure are age-related
      g. Assessment of jugular vein not required
      h. Assessment of temporal, brachial, popliteal, dorsalis pedis, and posterior tibial pulses not customary
   2. Geriatric
      a. Assess client comfort in supine position
      b. Heart rate slows with aging
      c. S3 is not normal in elderly clients
      d. Assessment of extremities for adequacy of circulation is vital
      e. Posterior tibial and dorsalis pedis pulses are difficult to palpate with aging
      f. Functional systolic murmurs increase with age; heard best at base or aortic area; requires referral
      g. Peripheral vessels may be tortuous and distended

diastolic → always pathological

Points to Remember

Although the cardiovascular system is internal, it can be assessed through external inspection, palpation, and auscultation.

Knowledge of the physiology of the cardiovascular system leads to knowledge of the heart sounds and their implications.

Thorough auscultation must be performed with the client in several positions and with both bell and diaphragm.

Assessment of edema and the integumentary system at the extremities are essential in a cardiovascular exam.

Glossary

Murmur—abnormal vibratory sounds produced by: a) increased flow through normal valves (functional murmur); b) forward flow through irregular or constricted valves; c) backward flow through incompetent valves

Precordium—the area of the chest over the heart and great vessels; contains visible anatomic landmarks used in cardiac assessment

Sinus arrhythmia—the acceleration of pulse rate during inspiration and deceleration during expiration; produced by impulses from the vagus nerve to the pacemaker; a normal finding

Thrill—abnormal flow of blood palpated as a rushing sensation; comparable to palpating the larynx of a purring cat

Breast and Axilla Assessment

Learning Objectives

After studying this section, the reader should be able to:

- Describe the major structures of the breast and their functions.

- Perform a breast exam on female and male clients.

- Understand the importance of client self-breast exam.

- Teach self-breast exam to client.

XII. Breast and Axilla Assessment

A. **External breast structures and functions** (see figure below)
   1. Breasts
      a. Glandular structures appended to the chest wall
      b. Produce milk after childbirth
      c. Are secondary sex organs; in women they respond to hormonal change at puberty, then monthly and at menopause

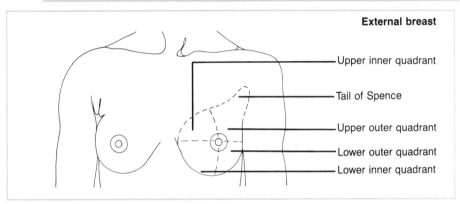

External breast

Upper inner quadrant

Tail of Spence

Upper outer quadrant

Lower outer quadrant

Lower inner quadrant

   2. Areola
      a. Pigmented area at tip of breast
      b. Montgomery's (sebaceous) glands will appear as papillae
      c. Hair follicles may be present at edge
   3. Nipple
      a. Pigmented area of erectile tissue at center of areola
      b. Area where milk ducts open

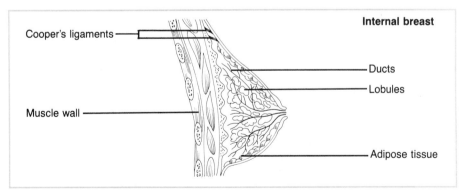

Internal breast

Cooper's ligaments

Ducts

Lobules

Muscle wall

Adipose tissue

B. **Internal structures and functions**
   1. Breast
      a. Glandular tissues: breast contains about 20 glandular lobes; 20 to 40 alveoli or lobules within each lobe contain milk-producing cells. Milk flows from lobes to storage ducts to duct openings in the nipple during nursing

   b. Fatty tissue: the majority of breast tissue; it surrounds and protects the
      glandular tissue
   c. Connective tissue: Cooper's (suspension) ligaments criss-cross the breast
      and attach to the chest wall muscles, supporting the breast
   d. Female glandular tissues change in consistency and sensitivity with
      monthly hormonal cycle; examination is best done within a week after
      menstruation ends
2. Associated lymph nodes in breast and axilla

look for dimpling usually tumor

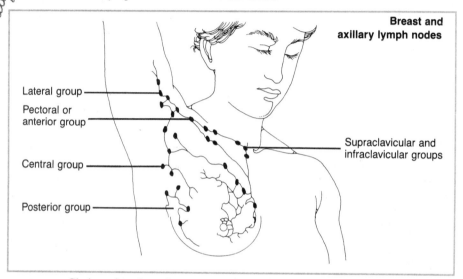

Breast and axillary lymph nodes

Lateral group

Pectoral or anterior group

Central group

Posterior group

Supraclavicular and infraclavicular groups

   a. Chains of nodes relevant to the breast are supra, sub, and infraclavicular;
      central and anterior axillary
   b. Lateral axillary (drains arm) and posterior axillary (drains parts of neck
      and thorax) are included because of their proximity
   c. Palpable nodes may indicate breast disease, including cancer

C. Inspection of the breast/axilla: procedure and normal findings
1. Examiner performs bilateral breast inspection with client in these positions:
   a. Sitting with arms at sides
   b. Sitting with arms above head
   c. Sitting with palms against hips or pressed together in front of body
   d. Sitting or standing, leaning forward, arms outstretched
2. Examiner performs unilateral breast inspection with client in supine position,
   places a towel under the shoulder of the side to be examined, and then tells
   client to place that arm under her head
3. Make the following assessments during breast inspection
   a. Skin should be smooth and move freely without puckering
   b. Striae and/or supernumerary nipples may be present
   c. Skin color should be uniform and match surrounding areas

    d. Moles or nevi should be longstanding and unchanged

    e. Breasts should be symmetrical or show slight, long-standing asymmetry; symmetry should be retained in all positions

    f. Size and contours should be bilaterally equal; no masses or retraction should be seen

    g. Areola should be symmetrical in size and placement

    h. Nipples should be symmetrically placed and pointing in same directions

    i. Nipples should show no cracks, crusting, or discharge

    j. Nipples should be everted or have long-standing inversion

    k. Axillae and clavicular areas should have appropriate hair distribution; no rash, ulceration, bulging, masses, or erythema

D. Palpation of the breasts/associated lymph nodes

  1. Examiner palpates breast and lymph nodes with palmar surface of fingers, the optimal technique for assessing masses

  2. Palpation for lymph nodes: procedure and normal findings

    a. Examiner performs with client sitting using light and deep palpation to assess all chains

    b. Examiner supports client's arm during axillary palpation to relax him/her and make palpation more effective

    c. Examiner palpates axilla with client's arm in several positions

    d. Nodes are seldom palpable in these chains

  3. Breast palpation: procedure and normal findings

    a. Examiner palpates each breast separately using a rotary motion; first lightly, then deeply

    b. Female client should be supine to spread the tissue

    c. Examiner palpates in either of two patterns (see figure); in concentric circles or inward from the periphery, like spokes on a wheel; regardless of pattern, consistency and thoroughness are vital

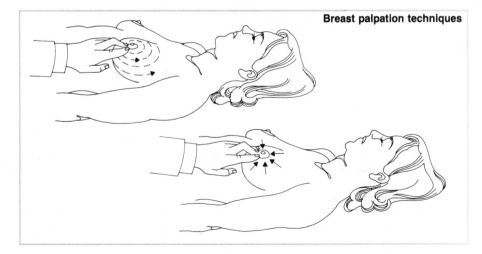

Breast palpation techniques

    d. Examiner adds bimanual palpation (support breast with one hand and palpate opposite side with other) in women with large breasts

    e. Examiner squeezes nipple following palpation of areola and nipple; no discharge should be produced

    f. Any mass should be described by location, size, mobility, surface characteristics, consistency, tenderness

    g. Healthy breast should be soft, elastic, with fine nodularity in glandular tissues; a firmer ridge of supporting tissue may be apparent from about 4:00 to 8:00, especially in larger breasts

E. Teaching the self-breast exam (SBE)

  1. SBE is the same as a professional exam, and can be taught during a clinical exam

  2. Points to remember:

    a. 90% of breast lumps are found first by clients

    b. SBE is conducted monthly, within first week after menstruation ends

    c. Breasts should be inspected in front of a mirror

    d. Many women feel increased palpation sensitivity in bath or shower

    e. Some women prefer their partner to do the SBE

    f. Regularity, consistent pattern, and thoroughness increase timely awareness of changes

F. Age and sex-related variations

  1. Pediatric

    a. Newborns may exhibit breast enlargement and nipple discharge from maternal hormones; lasts up to 3 months

    b. Inspection alone is adequate in pre-pubertal children without positive findings

    c. Adolescent breast development may be asymmetrical

    d. Breast tenderness may accompany development

    e. SBE should begin at menarche

    f. Development before age 9 requires evaluation

  2. Geriatric

    a. Breast size may decrease due to atrophy of glandular tissue and decrease in fat; skin may be wrinkled

    b. Supportive tissue softens, resulting in sagging

    c. Breast may feel stringy, granular, and/or nodular from glandular tissue change

    d. Post-menopausal women best remember monthly SBE by picking an easily remembered date (such as the birthdate)

    e. Men may exhibit an increase in fatty breast tissue

  3. Male breast

    a. Breast palpation can be done with client sitting and arms resting at sides

    b. The small band of breast tissue may not be palpable

    c. During puberty, males may exhibit normal gynecomastia

Points to Remember

Breasts are secondary sex organs: they respond to monthly hormonal changes and to developmental changes.

The most important part of breast assessment is teaching SBE to the client.

Breast assessment is important for males as well as females.

Caregivers must remember that breast examination can be a source of anxiety and embarrassment to many women.

Glossary

Erectile tissue—tissue that becomes swollen and rigid when filled with blood, especially sexual structures

Gynecomastia—excessive enlargement of male mammary glands

SBE (self breast exam)—self-care procedure with which clients can evaluate their own breasts for lesions, tenderness, or other changes

Tail of Spence—an extension of breast tissue from the upper outer quadrant of the breast into the axilla

Abdominal/Gastrointestinal Assessment

Learning Objectives

After studying this section, the reader should be able to:

• Locate major external anatomic landmarks of the abdomen.

• Identify placement of internal abdominal organs in relationship to landmarks.

• List major abdominal organs.

• Describe functions of major organs of GI system.

• List the sequence for performing abdominal assessments.

• Use inspection, auscultation, percussion and palpation to determine objective findings.

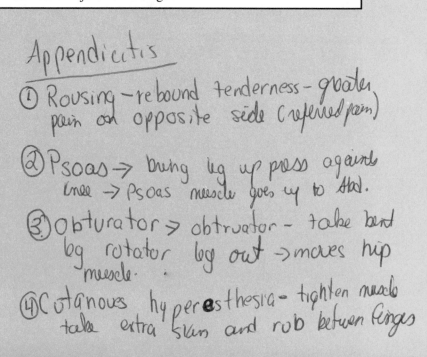

Appendicitis

① Rousing - rebound tenderness - greater pain on opposite side (referred pain)

② Psoas → bring leg up press against knee → Psoas muscle goes up to stat.

③ Obturator → obturator - take bent leg rotator leg out → moves hip muscle.

④ Cutanous hyperesthesia - tighten muscle take extra skin and rub between fingers

XIII. Abdominal/Gastrointestinal Assessment

A. External anatomic landmarks
1. Structures demarcating abdomen
    a. Xiphoid process
    b. Costal margin
    c. Rectus abdominus muscle
    d. Iliac crest
    e. Umbilicus
    f. Anterior-superior iliac spine
    g. Inguinal ligament
    h. Symphysis pubis
2. Imaginary quadrants demarcating abdomen (see figures below and on next page)
    a. Quadrants first divided by vertical line from sternum to pubic bone
    b. Second line drawn at right angle to first through umbilicus

B. Internal structures
1. Stomach (left upper quadrant)
    a. Begins at cardiac sphincter
    b. Empties into duodenum at pyloric sphincter
    c. Stores and digests food through hydrochloric acid and enzymatic secretion

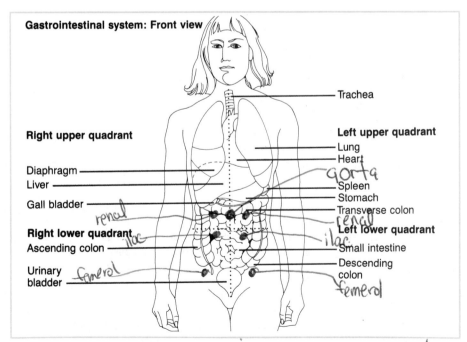

Gastrointestinal system: Front view

Trachea

Right upper quadrant

Left upper quadrant
Lung
Heart
aorta
Diaphragm
Liver
Spleen
Stomach
Gall bladder
Transverse colon
renal
renal
Right lower quadrant
iliac
Left lower quadrant
Ascending colon
iliac
Small intestine
Descending colon
Urinary bladder
femoral
femoral

Friction rub - over liver č G.C. Advance stages
(any liver inflamation)

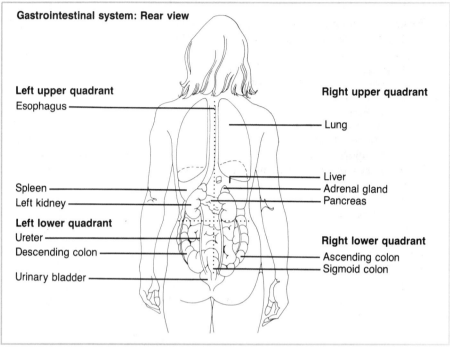

Gastrointestinal system: Rear view

Left upper quadrant
Esophagus

Right upper quadrant

Lung

Liver
Adrenal gland
Pancreas

Spleen
Left kidney

Left lower quadrant
Ureter

Right lower quadrant

Descending colon

Ascending colon
Sigmoid colon

Urinary bladder

2. Pancreas (left upper quadrant)
   a. Lies behind stomach
   b. Secretes endocrine hormones insulin and glucagon
3. Liver (right upper quadrant and left upper quadrant)
   a. Aids digestion of fat through bile secretion
   b. Produces plasma proteins
   c. Detoxifies plasma
   d. Aids breakdown of hemoglobin
4. Gallbladder (behind liver) stores bile
5. Spleen (left upper quadrant) produces and destroys hematologic elements
6. Small intestine (coiled in midabdomen; about 18 ft long)
   a. Duodenum, jejunum, ilium
   b. Villi in wall of intestine absorb proteins, fat, and carbohydrates
7. Large intestine
   a. Ascending colon (right upper and right lower quadrant)
   b. Descending colon (left upper and left lower quadrant)
   c. Transverse colon (right upper and left upper quadrant)
   d. Sigmoid colon (left lower quadrant)
   e. Cecum and appendix (right lower quadrant)
   f. Absorbs water and stores feces
8. Kidneys and adrenals (behind muscles of posterior abdominal wall)
   a. Right kidney is lower than left due to placement of liver

Arms must be @ side

    b. Only lower poles can be palpated
    c. Part of urinary system
    d. Maintain fluid and electrolyte balance
    e. Adrenals (on top of kidney): part of endocrine system

C. General Inspection: normal findings
   1. Skin — *Color, dry, scaley, bruised*
     a. Free from vascular lesions
     b. Free from jaundice
     c. Free from surgical scars
     d. Striae resulting from pregnancy or weight loss are pink or silver-white
   2. Contours — *Symmetry*
     a. Flat in well clients of proper weight
     b. Rounded in obese clients
     c. Scaphoid or concave in thin clients
     d. Symmetrical
     e. Free from umbilical or incisional hernias
   3. Movement
     a. Abdominal movement with respiration normal in males and children under age 7
     b. Absence of abdominal respiratory movement in males and young children indicates peritoneal irritation
     c. Visible right to left peristaltic movement seen in thin individuals

enlarged livers organs
masses.
Peristalasis (thin)
palsation.

D. Auscultation; performed before percussion and palpation because both can increase bowel motility and sounds: normal findings
   1. Peristaltic sounds
     a. Audible through diaphragm of stethoscope
     b. Occur every 5 to 15 seconds   *5-34/min.*
     c. High-pitched and gurgling in quality
     d. Peristalsis may be stimulated by gently flicking abdominal wall with finger
   2. Vascular sounds
     a. Audible with bell of stethoscope
     b. Audible over abdominal aorta
     c. Audible over renal arteries
     d. Audible over iliac arteries
     e. Free from murmurs
     f. Free from bruits
     g. Free from peritoneal friction rubs
     h. Venous hum normally heard over inferior vena cava

diastasis recti;
Abd muscle either
remain apart it indentation
or bulge

E. Percussion: normal findings
   1. Tympany
     a. Lower-pitched when percussed over gastric bubble
     b. High-pitched tympany over gas-filled bowel

finding landmarks
liver
stomach
spleen

borborygmi - hyperactive bowel sounds

2. Dullness
   a. Percussed over liver 6 to 12 cm in midclavicular line and 4 to 8 cm in midsternal line − liver
   b. Percussed over spleen sixth or ninth rib to 11th rib in left midaxillary line
   c. Shifting dullness heard over abdominal cavity in presence of ascites fluid
3. Indirect percussion
   a. Percussion over costo-vertebral junction elicits no pain over kidney area
   b. Fist percussion over liver elicits no liver pain

F. Palpation: normal findings
1. Light palpation; accomplished by fingertip exploration of all four quadrants
   a. No tenderness elicited
   b. No masses felt
   c. Organs should not be palpable
   d. Abdominal musculature should be free from tenderness or spasticity during expiration
2. Deep palpation; accomplished by bimanual method using two hands or by depressing abdomen with distal half of palmar surface of fingers: Normal findings
   a. Liver seldom palpable in adults
   b. Liver edge palpable in some persons; should have regular contour; sharp, non-tender, and felt no more than 2 cm below right costal margins
   c. Spleen not ordinarily palpable
   d. Kidney palpable only in thin clients or those with flaccid abdominal wall; right felt more often than left; should feel solid and firm
   e. Masses normally felt include: a full bladder at midline; pregnant uterus; colon filled with feces
   f. Deep palpation should elicit no pain
   g. Deep palpation should reveal no distention or ascites

G. Age and ethnic variations
1. Pediatric
   a. Abdomen larger than chest in children under age 4
   b. Contours should be rounded in pre-pubescent children
   c. Respiratory movement present in children under age 7
   d. Umbilical hernias present in some white children up until age 2
   e. Liver palpable 1 to 2 cm below costal margin in first year
   f. Spleen more easily palpated, but tip should not extend more than 1 cm below left costal margin
   g. Deep palpation should be done more gently in children
   h. Right to left peristaltic waves visible in infant
   i. Abdominal skin palpation can indicate child's state of hydration
2. Geriatric
   a. Palpation easier because abdominal wall is slacker
   b. Older clients have less pain with abdominal pathology

Points to Remember

Accurate examination of the abdomen requires knowledge of external landmarks and location of internal structures in relationship to landmarks.

To avoid stimulation of peristalsis, examination of the abdomen follows this sequence: inspection, auscultation, percussion, and palpation.

Liver dullness should extend from 6 to 12 cm in midclavicular line and 4 to 8 cm in midsternal line.

Splenic dullness should not extend beyond 10th rib.

The liver should not be palpable more than 2 cm below right costal margin.

The adult spleen should not be palpable.

Glossary

Ascites—accumulation of free fluid within abdominal cavity

Scaphoid abdomen—concave profile of abdomen in horizontal plane, sometimes indicative of malnutrition but can be seen normally in thin people

Stria (pl. striae)—a white line in skin caused by weakening of elastic tissue

liver

put on hand underneath and one on top.
liver take a deep breath
exhale → liver falls down.

spleen → under tenth rib
dullness - Abnormal sound
tympanny — normal sounds

Ascites

high pitch
top

tympani

dullness

Genitourinary (GU) Assessment

Learning Objectives

After studying this section, the reader should be able to:

• Describe the structures, functions and systems included in the genitourinary data base.

• Compare and contrast female and male anatomy and physiology.

• Perform a female genitourinary system exam, using inspection and palpation and including related lymphatic and anal assessments.

• Perform a male genitourinary system exam using inspection and palpation and including related lymphatic and anal assessments.

• Record findings of the genitourinary/lymph node/anal exam accurately and systematically.

XIV. Genitourinary (GU) Assessment

A. This data base includes the following systems and divisions

1. Lower excretory and reproductive systems (these are combined because of their anatomic proximity)
2. Adjacent lymphatic chains
3. The anus (part of the GI system; assessed here for convenience and because it is used in the GU examination)
4. Male and female systems (content is divided by sex, for ease of description and to facilitate caregiver review of the examination process)

B. External structures and functions: female

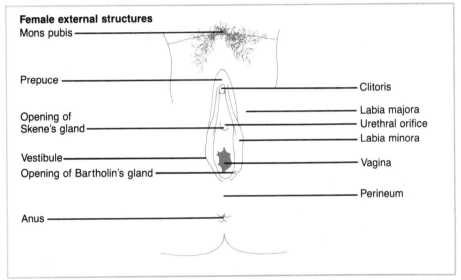

Female external structures
Mons pubis
Prepuce — Clitoris
Opening of Skene's gland — Labia majora / Urethral orifice / Labia minora
Vestibule — Vagina
Opening of Bartholin's gland
Perineum
Anus

1. Perineum: pelvic floor and associated structures, bounded by pubic symphysis, ischial tuberosities, and the coccyx
2. External genitalia, also known as vulva
   a. Clitoris: female erectile structure, homologous to penis
   b. Skene's glands: homologous to the male prostate
   c. Introitus: external orifice of the vagina
   d. Hymen: a protective membrane; may partly or wholly cover the introitus
   e. Bartholin's glands: source of mucus during sexual excitement
3. Anus: external voluntary sphincter of the large intestine

C. Internal structures and functions: female (see figure, next page)

1. Genitalia
   a. Vagina: a flexible muscular channel; it is also the birth canal
   b. Uterus: organ in which the fetus develops. Upper end is called the fundus and lower tubular part the cervix

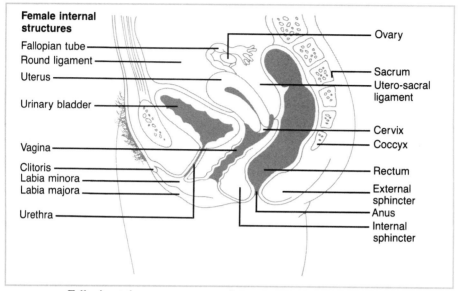

Female internal structures

Fallopian tube
Round ligament
Uterus
Urinary bladder
Vagina
Clitoris
Labia minora
Labia majora
Urethra

Ovary
Sacrum
Utero-sacral ligament
Cervix
Coccyx
Rectum
External sphincter
Anus
Internal sphincter

   c. Fallopian tubes: transport egg from ovary to uterus. The egg and sperm usually unite here

   d. Ovaries: the female gonads; they produce female hormones and grow and discharge ova

 2. Excretory structures

   a. Urethra: voluntarily excretes urine from the bladder

   b. Bladder: a storage sac for urine

 3. The anus and rectum

   a. Anus: voluntarily expels feces from the rectum

   b. Rectum: a receptacle for feces. Distension of the rectum sets up impulse that signals a need to move the bowels

 4. Related lymph nodes

   a. Horizontal inguinal chains: in groin. Drain external genitalia, perineum, anus, gluteus, lower abdominal wall

   b. Vertical inguinal chains: in upper, inner aspect of thigh. Drain legs, share some of above drainage areas

D. Inspection: female

 1. Client should be in dorsolithotomy position, draped, and made as comfortable as possible. She may place feet on table or in stirrups

 2. Genitalia: normal findings

   a. Hair should be dense, coarse, kinky, grows in an inverted triangular pattern on the mons and down sides of perineum

   b. Labia minora, vestibule and introitus should be moist

   c. No lesions, inflammation, masses, discharge, or odor should be present

   d. Vaginal wall should not prolapse into orifice

3. Anus: normal findings
   a. Circular area of increased pigmentation and coarse skin
   b. No tags, pouching, or fissures should be seen
4. Lymph nodes: normal findings
   a. No inflammation
   b. No visible nodes
5. Internal inspection with speculum: procedure and normal findings
   a. Examiner warms speculum before inserting; do not lubricate if Papanicolaou smear is to be obtained. Insert two fingers into introitus and press against posterior wall to relax vagina, then insert speculum at 45 degree downward angle
   b. Cervix should be midline, smooth, round, pink (bluish in pregnancy), about 2.5 cm diameter
   c. Cervix may have Nabothian cysts
   d. Os (cervical opening) should be small and round if nulliparous, slitlike if parous. Opening may be erythematous
   e. Os may contain creamy or clear, odorless mucous plug (especially at midcycle or just premenstrual)
   f. Walls should appear pink (bluish if premenstrual or pregnant), rugous, and moist as speculum is withdrawn
   g. Vagina may have thin, clear/cloudy, odorless discharge

E. Palpation: female
1. External genitalia: normal findings
   a. Perineal area should be soft; no masses or tenderness
   b. Palpation of Skene's and Bartholin's glands or milking urethra should produce no discharge or tenderness
   c. Perineum should be thick if nulliparous, thin if parous, when palpated between index finger and thumb
   d. Client can voluntarily constrict introitus around examining finger (more tightly if nulliparous); when bearing down against finger, no bulging or incontinence should result
2. Bimanual exam: procedure and normal findings
   a. Examiner inserts two fingers into vagina; it should be smooth and nontender
   b. With fingers at cervix, examiner places palmar surface of fingers of other hand on abdomen above pubis and press toward cervix; it should be firm, smooth, mobile, non-tender
   c. With gloved fingers in anterior fornix, examiner presses abdominal fingers downward more deeply; uterus should feel smooth, firm, have mobility, and exhibit no tenderness
   d. With gloved fingers in right or left fornix and abdominal fingers on same side, examiner slides fingers toward each other. Fallopian tube should not be palpable; ovary may be palpable and should be firm, smooth, mobile, tender

3. Recto-vaginal exam: procedure and normal findings
   a. Examiner should use new glove to prevent cross-contamination
   b. Examiner inserts index finger into vagina, middle finger into rectum and places other hand on abdomen. Palpate all rectal wall surfaces; they should be smooth, non-tender, without nodules or masses. Retro-flexed uterus may be palpable from rectum
   c. Withdraw rectal finger; sphincter should remain tight
4. Lymph nodes: normal findings
   a. Inguinal nodes should be small and firm or not palpable
   b. If palpable, they should be smooth, discrete, mobile, non-tender

F. Age-related variations: female
1. Pediatric
   a. Newborns may have engorged labia minora, erect clitoris, and sanguinous vaginal discharge from maternal hormones
   b. Genitalia growth in child is proportional to body size
   c. Internal vaginal examination unnecessary in healthy prepubertal females
   d. Urethral meatus may be adjacent to or slightly within introitus
   e. Periodic watery discharge may precede menarche by 1 to 2 years
2. Geriatric
   a. Vulvar hair becomes sparse, labia may shrink
   b. Vaginal wall becomes thin, atrophic, smoother, dry
   c. Vaginal canal shortens and narrows
   d. Perineal and sphincter tone decreases
   e. Cervix protrudes less in vagina, Nabothian cysts common

G. External structures and functions: male
1. Penis: the external male organ of excretion and copulation
   a. Shaft: body of the penis composed of corpus cavernosum and corpus spongiosum (erectile tissues)
   b. Glans penis or prepuce: end of the shaft; may be covered by foreskin or circumcised
2. Scrotum: pouch that supports testes, of dark, rugous skin
3. Anus: see female section

H. Internal structures and functions: male
1. Genitalia
   a. Penis: erectile organ to insert and ejaculate semen into the vagina
   b. Testes: male sex organ, produces both spermatozoa and testosterone. Sperm moves from seminiferous tubules of testicles into epididymis and from there to vas deferens. The spermatic cord, containing the vas, nerves, arteries, veins, and lymphatic vessels, passes through the inguinal canal to the abdominal cavity. It joins the seminal vesicle which secretes fluid to protect sperm. Cowper's gland also secretes protective fluid
   c. Prostate: heart-shaped gland lying beneath bladder and just anterior to rectum; secretes fluid to liquify sperm

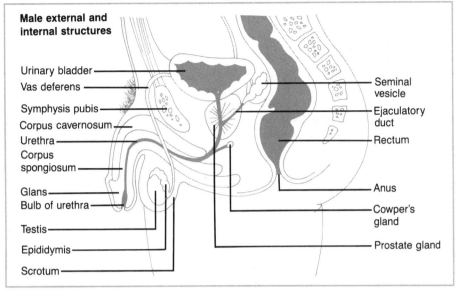

Male external and internal structures

Urinary bladder
Vas deferens
Symphysis pubis
Corpus cavernosum
Urethra
Corpus spongiosum
Glans
Bulb of urethra
Testis
Epididymis
Scrotum

Seminal vesicle
Ejaculatory duct
Rectum
Anus
Cowper's gland
Prostate gland

2. Excretory structures
   a. Urethra: as described in female section, but longer and carries semen as well as urine
   b. Bladder: see female section
3. Anus and rectum: see female section
4. Related lymph nodes: see female section

I. Inspection: male, normal findings

1. Pubic hair dense, coarse, curly, often with diamond-shaped distribution
2. Penis
   a. Dark, hairless, wrinkled
   b. Foreskin retracts easily, if not circumcised
   c. Urinary meatus centrally located with no discharge
   d. No inflammation, edema, scars, rashes, nodules
3. Scrotum
   a. Skin darker than surrounding skin, lies in loose folds
   b. Hair scant or absent
   c. Pendulous, with left side lower than right
   d. Not engorged, scarred, ulcerated, nodular, inflamed
   e. Does not transilluminate light if both testes present
4. Anus: see female section
5. Lymph: see female section

J. Palpation: male

1. Penis: normal findings
   a. Non-tender, smooth, with no masses or induration

  b. No erythema or discharge should be noted when client presses glans to open distal end of urethra

2. Scrotum: normal findings
   a. Skin should be thin, loose, non-tender
   b. One testis should be in each sack: equal in size, moveable, firm, rubbery, oval, moderately tender, smooth
   c. Epididymis should be on posterolateral surface of each testis; crescent-shaped, smooth, mobile, non-tender
   d. Vas deferens and spermatic cord: discretely palpable to inguinal ring, non-tender, mobile, smooth
   e. Scrotum should contain no additional contents

3. Inguinal ring: procedure and normal findings
   a. Examiner assesses for hernia with client standing
   b. Examiner uses index finger to follow spermatic cord up to inguinal ring
   c. When client bears down no mass will be felt

4. Femoral area: normal findings—no bulges should be felt when client bears down

5. Rectal exam with client lying on left side: procedure and normal findings
   a. Examiner inserts lubricated finger (after client bears down)
   b. Sphincter should be evenly tight
   c. Rectal walls smooth without nodules, masses, tenderness
   d. Prostate palpated at anterior surface; should be about 4 cm diameter, firm, smooth, with palpable sulcus (groove); non-tender, with no enlargement, irregularity, or masses
   e. Any stool present on withdrawn finger should be brown

6. Lymph nodes: as in female

K. Age-related variations: male

1. Pediatric
   a. Penis and scrotum are proportionate to body size before puberty; are disproprotionately large in early puberty
   b. Cremasteric reflex very active in infants and young boys; reflexive retraction of the testis may give appearance of an undescended testicle
   c. Pubertal boys should be taught how to do self testicular exam: to demonstrate, palpate each testis by rolling it between thumb and first two fingers; examine for lumps, tenderness, contour, consistency, and mobility

2. Geriatric
   a. Pubic hair thins and grays
   b. Slight testicular atrophy may occur
   c. Prostate gland may enlarge, patient may have nocturnal urinary frequency
   d. Scrotal sac may elongate

Points to Remember

Consider the client's potential discomfort with this area of the physical exam. Be aware of your own feelings.

Conduct exam efficiently and without interruption to minimize time exposed or (for females) in stirrups.

Teach testicular self exam to all males at puberty or older.

Examine anus and rectum at this time because of their close proximity and relationship to the prostate and uterus.

Glossary

Dorsolithotomy position—client lying on back with thighs flexed upon abdomen and lower legs abducted toward thighs; commonly used for female pelvic exams

Fornix (pl. fornices)—the recess formed by the protrusion of the cervix into the vagina

Groin—the depression between the thigh and the trunk; the inguinal region

Nabothian cysts—small, round, raised, yellowish sebaceous cysts formed by the Nabothian glands of the cervix

Ruga (pl. rugae)—a fold or crease in epithelium

Musculoskeletal Assessment

Learning Objectives

After studying this section, the reader should be able to:

- Describe the major components of the musculoskeletal system.

- Define seven types of joint motion.

- Use inspection and palpation to examine the musculo-skeletal system.

- Record pertinent objective findings from the exam.

long — legs, arms

short - feet, finger,

flat → sternum, ribs
       scula skull

irregular → spine
            wrist
            ankles

periosteum - sqt membrane
             blood flow

cortex (hard)

spongey (cancellous)

medullary canal
(nutrients)

600 muscle
voluntary - skeletal - you give it
involuntary - blood vessels - bronchi
              GI - uterus
heart — myocardium

Bursa — fluid sacs
        that reduce friction

XV. Musculoskeletal Assessment

A. Major components of the musculoskeletal system
1. Bones: 206   *mobility   mineral storage*
   a. Support and protect other tissues
   b. Contain hematopoietic (myeloid) tissue, or marrow, which produces red blood cells
   c. Axial skeleton: bones of head, ribs, and vertebral column   *heat production*
   d. Appendicular skeleton: shoulders, pelvis, and extremities
2. Cartilage
   a. Allows full joint movements
   b. Protects articulating surfaces of bones
3. Connective tissue
   a. Muscles: principal organs of movement
   b. Tendons: tough, fibrous portions of muscle that join muscle to bone
   c. Ligaments: tough, fibrous bands that join bone to bone
4. Synovial joint: type of movable joint (see figure below)
   a. Joint space: cavity between bone ends, permits free movement
   b. Joint capsule: sac-like envelope enclosing the cavity of a synovial joint
   c. Synovial membrane: secretes synovial fluid for lubrication of joints

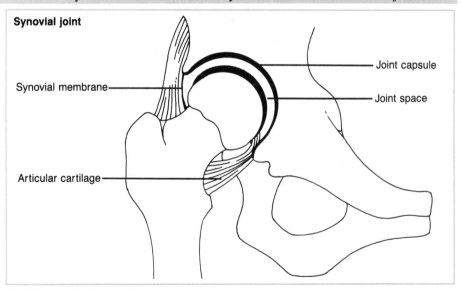

Synovial joint

Synovial membrane

Articular cartilage

Joint capsule

Joint space

B. Types of joint motion
1. Flexion: bending a limb, lessening the joint angle
2. Extension: straightening a limb, increasing the joint angle
3. Abduction: moving a limb away from midline of body
4. Adduction: moving a limb toward the central axis of the body
5. Internal rotation: turning a body part inward toward central axis of body
6. External rotation: turning a body part away from midline
7. Circumduction: moving a limb in circular fashion

[handwritten: muscle proximal to joint enter a pull over joint and cause a movement]

C. Inspection of musculoskeletal system
1. General: normal findings
   a. Gross deformities should be absent
   b. Symmetry of body parts should be evident
   c. Posture should be straight
   d. Alignment of body should be even

[handwritten: guarding → don't move]

RANGE OF MOTION*

Joint	Motion	Approximate Measurement
Temporomandibular	Open wide (active) Mandible forward	Able to insert three fingers Top teeth behind lower teeth
Neck	Flexion Extension Rotation	45° 55° 70°
Trunk	Flexion Extension Rotation Lateral bending	70-90° 30° standing 20° prone 30-45° 35°
Shoulder	Forward flexion (arm straight) Backward extension (arm straight) Horizontal extension (arm straight) Horizontal flexion (arm straight) Abduction (arm straight) Adduction (arm straight) Abduction† Adduction†	180° 50-60° 130° 40° 180° 45-50° 90° 90°
Elbow	Flexion Extension Hyperextension Supination Pronation	150° 150° 0-15° 90° 90°
Wrist	Flexion Extension Radial deviation Ulnar deviation	80-90° 70° ± 20° 30°-50°
Fingers Metacarpophalangeal joints	Flexion Extension Abduction Adduction	90° 30-45° 20° between fingers Fingers should touch
Proximal interphalangeal joints	Flexion Extension	100-200° 0°
Distal interphalangeal joints	Flexion Extension	80-90° 20°
Thumb	Flexion Extension	Transpalmar abduction Able to touch tip of thumb to base of little finger and then extend away from the palm 50° between thumb and index finger

Reprinted with permission from Block, Gloria J., et al. *Health Assessment for Professional Nursing: A Developmental Approach*, Appleton & Lange, 1981.

RANGE OF MOTION* continued

Joint	Motion	Approximate Measurement
Thumb (continued) Metacarpophalangeal joint	Flexion Extension	50°
Interphalangeal joint	Flexion Extension	90° 20°
Palmar	Abduction Adduction	70° 70°
Opposition	Able to touch each fingertip with tip of thumb	
Hip	Flexion Knee flexed Knee straight Extension (prone) Abduction Adduction Internal rotation External rotation	110-120° 90° or less 30° or less 45-50° 20-30° 35-40° 45°
Knee	Flexion Extension (hyper) Internal rotation External rotation	120-130° 10-15° 10° 10°
Ankle and foot	Extension (dorsiflexion) Flexion (plantar flexion) Inversion (passive), hind foot Eversion (passive), hind foot Abduction, forefoot Adduction, forefoot	20° 45-50° 5° 5° 10° 20°
Toes First metatarsophalangeal joint	Flexion (active) Extension (active)	45° 70-90°
Interphalangeal joints	Distal Flexion Extension	60° 30°
	Proximal Flexion Extension	35° 0°
Metatarsophalangeal joints	Flexion Extension	40° 40°
Toe spread	Abduction/adduction	Degrees vary

*Active unless otherwise stated. †Elbow held at side and flexed.

    e. Slope of spine should reveal normal curves   *facial expression*
    f. Involuntary movement should be absent
    g. Gait should be smooth
  2. Active range of motion (ROM): upper body muscles and joints (see table above and on previous page for ROM norms)
    a. Temporomandibular joint

    b. Neck
    c. Trunk
    d. Shoulder
    e. Elbow
    f. Wrist
    g. Fingers
    h. Thumb
    i. Palms
  3. Active range of motion should be within norms: lower body (see table on p. 110-111).
    a. Hip
    b. Knee
    c. Ankle
    d. Foot
    e. Toes
  4. No swelling of joints or muscles should be visible
  5. No inflammation should be visible
  6. No pain with active range of motion should be present
  7. Normal curve of spine should be visible
    a. No scoliosis, i.e., no deviation of thoracic curve when client bends at the waist
    b. No lordosis, i.e., no increased concavity of lumbar spine
  8. Posterior thorax should be without deformity
    a. Scapulae equal
    b. Pelvis symmetrical
  9. Measurement with tape measure
    a. Length of extremities should be equal
    b. Muscle mass should be symmetrical

D. Palpation: normal findings
  1. No swelling — temperature change
  2. No tenderness   heat
  3. No changes in normal shape
  4. No deformity
  5. Muscle tone should be equal bilaterally with movement
  6. Symmetrical consistency in muscle texture
  7. No involuntary contractions or twitching
  8. Passive range of motion: procedure and normal findings
    a. Examiner moves all joints through range of motion
    b. No pain
    c. No crepitus
    d. No loose bodies
    e. No fluid
    f. No weakness
  9. Assessment of muscle strength: procedures
    a. Examiner systematically tests muscle group resistance from head to toe

    b. Examiner tries to open client's shut eyes

    c. Examiner palpates cheeks while client puffs them

    d. Examiner palpates resistance to neck extension

    e. Examiner tries to push arms down while client raises them, a test of deltoid muscle strength

    f. Client extends arms while examiner tries to push them downward

    g. Client extends arms while examiner tries to flex them, a test of tricep strength

    h. Client tries to resist examiner's flexion of wrist, a test of wrist and finger muscles

    i. Client shakes both hands of examiner at the same time

    j. Examiner tries to hold down extended leg while client raises it, an assessment of hip muscles

    k. Client sits and alternately crosses legs to assess hamstring, gluteal and abductor muscles

    l. Client extends leg against resistance to assess quadriceps

    m. Client presses foot and toe against examiner's hands to assess foot and ankle muscles

    n. Client walks on toes

    o. Client walks on heels

    p. Client hops

E. Age and ethnic considerations

  1. Pediatric

    a. Observe for torticollis; head tilts to one side from swelling of sternocleidomastoid muscle

    b. Observe for foot deformities, such as calcaneus and equinus, in neonate by checking resistance of foot to manipulation during range of motion

    c. Assess symmetry of gluteal folds for congenital hip dislocation

    d. Test for Ortolani's sign on neonate

    e. Screen school-aged and adolescent children for scoliosis

    f. Screen toddlers for tibial torsion, bow legs (varus deviation), or knock knees (valgus deviation)

  2. Geriatric

    a. Normal reduction of muscle mass, but not a loss of strength

    b. Presence of Heberden's nodes; bony overgrowth in distal finger joints related to osteoarthritis

    c. Kyphosis of spine related to osteoporosis

  3. Ethnic considerations

    a. Normal lumbar curves more pronounced in black children

    b. Peroneus muscle of foot may be decreased in size or absent in Blacks and Native Americans

Points to Remember

The major components of the musculoskeletal system are bones, joints, tendons, ligaments, and muscles.

Inspection of the musculoskeletal system includes observing for obvious deformity, abnormality in gait, or limitation in active range of motion.

Palpation of the musculoskeletal system includes feeling for deformity, tenderness, swelling, effusion, muscle tone, limitation in passive range of motion, and decrease in muscle strength against resistance.

Additional screenings of the musculoskeletal system are performed in pediatric examination.

Glossary

Calcaneus—congenital deformity of foot that causes dorsiflexion

Equinus—congenital deformity of foot that causes plantar flexion

Valgus—deviation of a body part inward; e.g., knock-knee

Varus—deviation of a body part away from the midline; e.g., bowleg

hx
overall strength and ability
gait -
cordination
Abnormal muscle twitching
family hx - gout - arthritis
problems c̄ hands or feet
deformity
edema
weakness

Integumentary Assessment

Learning Objectives

After studying this section, the reader should be able to:

- Identify the structures and functions of the integument.

- Use inspection to identify normal objective findings.

- Use palpation to identify normal objective findings.

- Describe lesions on the integument.

- Record objective data related to the integument.

XVI. Integumentary Assessment

A. Structures of the integument and their functions
   1. Layers of the skin

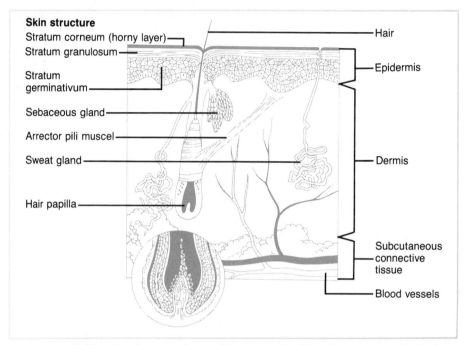

Skin structure
Stratum corneum (horny layer) — Hair
Stratum granulosum —
Stratum germinativum — Epidermis
Sebaceous gland —
Arrector pili muscel —
Sweat gland — Dermis
Hair papilla —
Subcutaneous connective tissue
Blood vessels

   a. Epidermis: the outer layer of keratinized cells and the inner cellular layer where melanin and keratin are formed
   b. Dermis: middle layer containing blood vessels, sebaceous glands, and some hair follicles
   c. Subcutaneous tissue: contains fat, sebaceous glands, and remainder of hair follicles
   2. Epidermal appendages
   a. Hair
   b. Nails
   c. Eccrine sweat glands; are widely distributed
   d. Apocrine sweat glands; open into hair follicles in axillary and genital areas
   e. Sebaceous glands; produce sebum
   3. Functions of skin and epidermal appendages
   a. Barrier to water and electrolyte loss
   b. Regulation of body heat
   c. Sensory organ for touch, temperature, and pain
   d. Production of protective skin film by eccrine and sebaceous glands
   e. Participation in production of vitamin D
   f. Wound repair

B. Inspection of skin
1. General inspection
   a. Use indirect natural lighting when possible
   b. Compare symmetrical anatomical areas
2. Inspection of color: normal findings
   a. Color varies with race
   b. Color of highly vascular areas such as cheeks and flexor surfaces vary with temperature changes
   c. Normal color is whitish pink or shades of brown, depending on race
   d. Cyanosis, pallor, jaundice, or erythema can indicate systemic disease

C. Palpation: normal findings
1. Temperature: warm but not hot
2. Moisture: varies with body part and activity
3. Texture: fineness or coarseness of skin
4. Turgor: elasticity; skin should return to normal shape when picked up and released

D. Inspection and palpation of epidermal appendages: hair and nails
1. Hair
   a. Note quantity
   b. Note distribution: female versus male
   c. Note color: varies with age
   d. Note texture: soft, smooth
2. Nails: normal findings
   a. Color: white lunula, semi-transparent nail plate
   b. Contour: rectangular with dorsal convexity
   c. Thickness: 0.3 to 0.65 mm
   d. Tenderness: normally non-tender to palpation

E. Description and classification of skin lesions
1. Types of lesions
   a. Primary: result from external or internal environment change; e.g., pustule
   b. Secondary: result from modification in a primary lesion; e.g., ulcer
2. Types of primary lesions
   a. Macule: 1 cm or less; change in skin color without elevation; area less than 1 cm in patch; e.g., freckle
   b. Papule: solid elevated area greater than 1 cm; larger variety of same lesions occur in a plaque
   c. Nodule: 0.5 to 2 cm lesion in dermal layer, e.g., wart; greater than 2-cm lesion is tumor
   d. Wheal: irregular, transient area of local skin edema; e.g., hive or mosquito bite
   e. Vesicle: 0.5 cm superficial elevation filled with serous fluid, e.g., herpes simplex; area greater than 0.5 cm is a bullae; e.g., second degree burn
   f. Pustule: pus-filled elevation; e.g., acne

3. Types of secondary lesions
   a. Erosion: loss of superficial epidermis; e.g., moist area after rupture of a vesicle
   b. Fissure: deep linear break in skin extending to dermis
   c. Crust: formed when serum, blood, or exudate dries on the skin; e.g., impetigo
   d. Scale: thin flakes of shedding epidermis; e.g., dandruff
   e. Scar: replacement of destroyed tissue by fibrous tissue
4. Types of shapes or configurations
   a. Round
   b. Linear
   c. Annular
   d. Grouped
5. Color
6. Location and distribution

F. Age and ethnic variations
1. Pediatric
   a. Neonates may have milia over nose and checks; these are small white papules caused by plugging of sebaceous glands
   b. Neonates often have "stork bites" or nevus flumus; these are small red macular patches over occiput, forehead, and upper eyelids
   c. Adolescents frequently have pustules and blackheads that occur with proliferation of sweat and sebaceous glands during puberty
2. Geriatric
   a. Skin thins, becomes less elastic
   b. Hair growth is scant
   c. Small scarlet vascular lesions (cherry angiomas) called senile telangiectasia are present from middle age onward
   d. Brown melanotic deposits, called age spots, are common
   e. Cutaneous skin tags, called acrochordons, are common; flesh-colored, soft, and pedunculated
3. Ethnic
   a. Brown- or black-skinned children have blue, irregularly shaped flat areas over sacrum and buttocks called mongolian spots; sometimes mistaken for bruises
   b. Abnormal color changes in dark-skinned persons are difficult to assess; pallor in black-skinned people may be ashen gray
   c. Cyanosis is best detected at least pigmented areas such as lips and oral mucosa in dark-skinned persons
   d. Jaundice in dark-skinned persons should be inspected with examination of hard palate
   e. Flushing as with fever is best inspected at the tips of the ears in dark-skinned individuals
   f. Normal shedding of the epidermal layer of dark-skinned individuals may appear to the inexperienced examiner as "dirt"

Points to Remember

The skin serves as a barrier to injury and regulates fluid balance through evaporation.

Hair and nails are epidermal appendages.

Color and appearance of skin, hair, and nails provides evidence of nutritional and health status.

Color and temperature in dark-skinned individuals is assessed in less-pigmented areas of the body.

Skin lesions are described in terms of type, color, location, configuration, and distribution.

Glossary

Apocrine glands—sweat glands found in axillary and genital regions

Cherry angioma—cherry-red vascular papules associated with normal aging or liver disease

Eccrine glands—widely distributed sweat glands

Keratin—outermost epidermal layer of dead cells

Melanin—skin and hair pigment formed by cells in epidermal layer

Sebum—oily substance produced by sebaceous glands to lubricate skin surface

Neurologic Assessment

Learning Objectives

After studying this section, the reader should be able to:

• Describe the basic structures and functions of the central and peripheral nervous system.

• List the major parts of the neurologic exam and what part of the nervous system each assesses.

• Perform a neurologic exam.

• Explain why some parts of the neurologic exam are performed elsewhere in a complete health exam. List those parts.

• Record the findings from the neurologic exam.

XVII. Neurologic Assessment

A. **Nervous system structures and functions: consists of brain, spinal cord, and peripheral nervous system. This complex communication and coordination system controls the body's adjustment and responses to internal and external stimuli.**

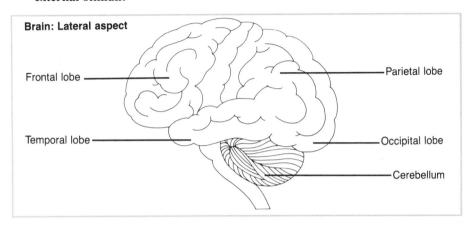

Brain: Lateral aspect

Frontal lobe

Parietal lobe

Temporal lobe

Occipital lobe

Cerebellum

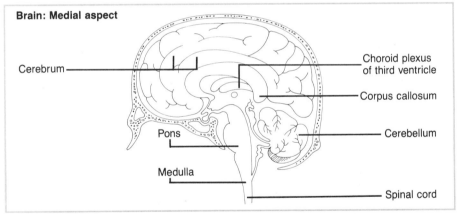

Brain: Medial aspect

Cerebrum

Choroid plexus of third ventricle

Corpus callosum

Pons

Cerebellum

Medulla

Spinal cord

1. Cerebrum: location of mental functioning; storehouse of information; area where motor and sensory data are interpreted
    a. Frontal lobes: largest areas of cerebrum; responsible for conscious thought, regulation of behavior and judgment, changes in mood/personality, voluntary movement
    b. Parietal lobes: responsible for perception of sensation, proprioception, pain, temperature, touch, speech organization, speech interpretation
    c. Temporal lobes: responsible for understanding speech, conscious memory, interpretation of hearing, smell (CN I), and taste, and some visual interpretation
    d. Occipital lobes: control most visual functioning (CN II)

2. Thalamus and hypothalamus: not amenable to neurologic assessment; affect autonomic and hormonal functions
3. Cerebellum: connected and related in function to cerebrum and brainstem; interprets and controls posture, equilibrium, voluntary muscle coordination and tone
4. Brainstem: controls reflex, autonomic, voluntary functions
   a. Midbrain contains center for visual reflexes (cranial nerves III, IV)
   b. Pons contains nerve nuclei for cranial nerves (CN) V, VI, VII, VIII
   c. Medulla contains nerve nuclei for CN IX, X, XI, XII as well as autonomic centers for respiration, circulation, and blood pressure
5. Cranial nerves (see above for associated brain center): peripheral nerves that arise within skull; they serve the head and neck and have sensory and/or motor functions

CRANIAL NERVE FUNCTIONS

Name and number of cranial nerve	Motor (m) or sensory (s) origin	Function or area of innervation
CN I (olfactory)	S	Smell
CN II (optic)	S	Vision
CN III (oculomotor)	M	Pupillary constriction; extraocular muscles
CN IV (trochlear)	M	Extraocular muscles
CN V (trigeminal)	S	Face and scalp; three divisions: ophthalmic, maxillary, andibular
	M	Mandibular muscles
CN VI (abducens)	M	Lateral deviation of eye
CN VII (facial)	S	Taste: anterior two-thirds of tongue
	M	Facial muscles: forehead, mouth, outer ear
CN VIII (acoustic)	S	Hearing, balance
CN IX (glossopharyngeal)	S	Taste: rear third of tongue
	M	Pharynx: swallowing, gagging
CN X (vagus)	S	Larynx, pharynx, esophagus
	M	Pharynx, larynx
CN XI (spinal accessory)	M	Muscles: sternocleidomastoid, trapezius
CN XII (hypoglossal)	M	Tongue

6. Spinal nerves
   a. There are 31 pairs of spinal nerves: 8 cervical, 12 thoracic, 5 lumbar, 5 sacral, 1 coccygeal
   b. Each nerve contains dorsal and ventral branches and has afferent and efferent components
   c. Spinal nerves can be assessed for motor function (muscle tone, strength and movement), sensory function (tactile, vibration, pain, temperature) and reflex status (requiring both afferent and efferent functioning)

B. **Neurologic screening**
   1. In the absence of neurologically signifiant history, presenting complaint, and/or related positive physical exam findings, a neurologic screening exam provides adequate data for assessment of neurologic health
   *2. The screening exam comprises those items preceded by an asterisk

*Denotes element of a neurologic screening examination.

C. Cerebral functioning

1. Mental status: tested during general objective assessment section of exam (see Section V) and while gathering other data. Areas to be assessed are:
   *a. Cognitive: level of consciousness, orientation, memory (immediate, recent, remote), attention/concentration, judgment, abstract reasoning, calculation ability
   *b. Emotional: appropriate appearance and behavior, affect, mood
   *c. Thought process/content: appropriate and realistic perceptions and thoughts
2. Specific cortical functions
   a. Sensory recognition: client can identify familiar sounds (auditory recognition), objects by sight (visual recognition), and objects by touch (tactile recognition). Client knows right from left and identifies body parts (body relationship recognition)
   *b. Skilled motor ability: client can carry out purposive, multipart activity (requires understanding, remembering, and integrating instructions, and having requisite motor skills)
   *c. Skilled speech and language functions: client can answer questions appropriately (auditory-receptive integration), carry on relevant conversation (expressive speaking function), read a sentence and interpret its meaning (visual-receptive integration), and write with eyes open, then closed (expressive writing)

D. Cranial nerves: assessment for nerves described on previous page (most of these assessments are covered in appropriate body system): normal findings

1. I: client can identify a variety of smells
*2. II: client has visual acuity, full visual fields; fundoscopic exam reveals no pathology
*3. III, IV, VI: client follows to six cardinal positions of gaze; PERRLA is unremarkable, has no nystagmus, no ptosis
*4. V: client clenches teeth with firm bilateral pressure; has no lateral jaw deviation with mouth open; feels cotton wisp on forehead, cheek, and chin; differentiates sharp/dull sensation on face; blinks when cotton is touched to each cornea
*5. VII: client has facial symmetry, can symmetrically raise eyebrows and grimace; shut eyes tightly; identify sweet, salt, sour on anterior tongue
*6. VIII: client can hear whisper at 1 ft to 2 ft (0.3 to 0.6 m), watch tick at 1″ to 2″ (2.5 to 5 cm), does not lateralize Weber test, and hears AC>BC in Rinne test
*7. IX, X: client speaks and swallows without hoarseness; palate and uvula rise symmetrically with "Ah"; has bilateral gag reflex
*8. XI: client demonstrates resistance to head turning and can shrug against resistance
*9. XII: client can stick tongue out, move it from side to side and push it strongly against resistance

*Denotes element of a neurologic screening examination.

E. Cerebellar functioning
1. Gross motor and balance testing (client standing): normal findings
   a. Client has smooth, coordinated gait
   *b. Client can balance with hands outstretched and eyes open, then closed (Romberg test); (note: support client if he/she begins to fall)
   c. Client can walk on tiptoes, then on heels
   *d. Client can do heel to toe walk
   e. Client can balance on one foot, then the other
2. Fine motor of upper extremities (client seated): normal findings
   *a. Client can rapidly touch alternating index fingers to nose, first with eyes open, then closed
   b. Client can rapidly alternate touching finger to own nose, then to examiner's finger (examiner moves her/his finger each time); assessed with each hand
3. Fine motor of lower extremities (client seated): normal findings
   *a. Client can run each heel smoothly down opposite shin
   b. Client can make a figure 8 in the air with each foot

F. Motor system functioning—See Musculoskeletal Assessment Section XV

G. Sensory system function (with client's eyes closed): normal findings
1. Primary sensory: note symmetry of response and test a number of areas on body
   *a. Superficial tactile: client identifies spot touched with cotton wisp
   *b. Superficial pain: identifies spot touched with pin
   c. Temperature: differentiates hot and cold test tubes
   d. Vibration: identifies when a vibrating tuning fork is touched to a bony prominence
   e. Position sense: can describe motion and final position after fingers and toes are passively moved
2. Discriminatory sensation: always note symmetry
   a. Stereognosis: client identifies familiar objects in hand
   *b. Graphesthesia: identifies numbers drawn on each palm
   c. Two point discrimination: discriminates between being touched by one or two sharp objects in various parts of the body (note distances used between objects)

H. Reflexes
1. Principles of testing reflexes
   a. Apply stimulus to both sides with same intensity
   b. Ensure that part to be tested is relaxed
   c. Rate rapidity and strength of contraction, and compare bilaterally. Use stick figure to locate and rate.

*Denotes element of a neurologic screening examination.

2. Rating scale for reflexes
   a. 0: absent
   b. 1+ (or +): minimal, sluggish
   c. 2+ (or ++): brisk (normal)
   d. 3+ (or +++): brisker
   e. 4+ (or ++++): very brisk, hyperreactive, may exhibit clonus
3. Deep tendon reflexes: tap tendon smartly, causing sudden tendon stretching and evoking a contractile response of muscle
   a. Tendons and locations: triceps (above olecrenon process), biceps (in fossa of bent elbow), brachioradialis (proximal to styloid process of elbow), patellar (below patella), and achilles (above heel)
   b. Responses will be brisk and bilaterally equal
   *c. For screening, test only patellar reflex
4. Superficial reflexes: stroke skin lightly with sharp object, resulting in visible muscle contraction
   a. Areas tested and expected results: upper and lower abdominal (umbilicus moves up or down toward area being stroked); cremasteric (scrotum elevates); plantar surface (toes flex); gluteus (skin tenses)
   b. Responses will be brisk and bilaterally equal
   *c. For screening, test only abdominal reflex

I. Age-related variations

1. Pediatric: each developmental stage from birth to age 5 has its own neurologic assessment. Tests described in this section are appropriate for school-aged children unless intellectually or emotionally immature. Some considerations for younger children follow; consult a pediatric text for definitive assessment guides below age 5
   a. Infants are born with necessary primitive reflexes that decline during normal development and are replaced by higher, more integrated motor responses. These are assessed for appropriate presence or absence and for symmetry. A few well known examples are: sucking (present to age 3 months), moro (to age 3 or 4 months), and palmar grasp (to 6 months). Babinski's reflex is normal to about age 18 months
   b. A developmental screening tool such as the Denver Developmental Screening Test (DDST) provides a standardized guide to fine and gross motor, language, and personal-social development of children from birth to age 5
2. Geriatric
   a. Response time may slow with aging
   b. Senses of smell and taste may diminish
   c. Sensations and reflexes in feet and ankles may diminish
   d. Response to pain stimuli may decrease
   e. Other sensory and motor deficits may have non-neurologic causes, but can confuse responses to neurologic testing; e.g., the effect of cataracts on visual acuity

*Denotes element of a neurologic screening examination.

Points to Remember

A complete neurologic exam takes 2 to 3 hours. The screening assessment provides an adequate picture in the absence of significant history or other positive findings.

The neurologic screening depends on developmental level. Screening and expectations at each pediatric age will vary widely. A pediatric text is required to perform a specific age-related neurologic exam.

Much of the neurologic system data is gathered and recorded while assessing other systems; the practitioner must sort out pertinent data and conceptualize neurologic components in an integrated way.

The neurologic system coordinates and controls all other systems; it affects the entire body in complex and significant ways.

Glossary

Afferent—carrying toward the center from the periphery, centripetal

Autonomic—working without conscious or voluntary control

Efferent—carrying away from the center twoard the periphery; centrifugal

Index

Notes

Notes

Notes

Notes

Notes

Notes

Notes

Notes

Notes

Notes

Notes

Notes

Notes

Notes

Notes